Nursing Home Social Work Research

This book focuses on the characteristics, roles, and training needs of social service delivery providers in leadership roles in U.S. nursing facilities. The chapters in this volume explore a range of issues salient to nursing home social workers and social work practices such as realistic staffing ratios, qualification levels, dementia training needs, involvement in care transitions and admissions, and barriers to psychosocial care. This book also addresses the Social Service Directors' involvement in and preparation for disaster care planning, suicide risk management, and serious mental illness.

This edited collection will greatly benefit students, academics, and researchers in nursing, psychology, health, and social work. The chapters in this book were originally published as a special issue of the *Journal of Gerontological Social Work*.

Robin Bonifas is Professor and Chair of the Social Work Department at Indiana State University, Terre Haute, USA. She has over 15 years' experience working with older adults in long-term care and inpatient psychiatric settings. She is John A. Hartford Faculty Scholar and Editor-in-Chief of the *Journal of Gerontological Social Work*.

Mercedes Bern-Klug is Professor at the School of Social Work at the University of Iowa, USA. She specializes in gerontology, with a focus on long-term services, and supports for older persons and persons with disabilities. She conducts research on how social workers and other health care providers can support older adults and their family members with the psychosocial implications of medical decision-making in long-term care settings.

Nursing Home Social Work Research

Edited by
Robin Bonifas and Mercedes Bern-Klug

Routledge
Taylor & Francis Group

LONDON AND NEW YORK

First published 2024
by Routledge
4 Park Square, Milton Park, Abingdon, Oxon, OX14 4RN

and by Routledge
605 Third Avenue, New York, NY 10158

Routledge is an imprint of the Taylor & Francis Group, an informa business

British Library Cataloguing-in-Publication Data
A catalogue record for this book is available from the British Library

ISBN13: 978-1-032-50899-3 (hbk)
ISBN13: 978-1-032-50900-6 (pbk)
ISBN13: 978-1-003-40023-3 (ebk)

DOI: 10.4324/9781003400233

Typeset in Minion Pro
by codeMantra

Publisher's Note
The publisher accepts responsibility for any inconsistencies that may have arisen during the conversion of this book from journal articles to book chapters, namely the inclusion of journal terminology.

Disclaimer
Every effort has been made to contact copyright holders for their permission to reprint material in this book. The publishers would be grateful to hear from any copyright holder who is not here acknowledged and will undertake to rectify any errors or omissions in future editions of this book.

Contents

Citation Information   vii

Notes on Contributors   ix

Preface: Home is where you are known, comfortable, safe, and feel a sense of control   xi
Mercedes Bern-Klug

Introduction: Nursing Home Social Services Research   1
Robin P. Bonifas

1   About a Third of Nursing Home Social Services Directors Have Earned a Social Work Degree and License   3
Mercedes Bern-Klug, Kevin M. Smith, Amy Restorick Roberts, Nancy Kusmaul, Denise Gammonley, Paige Hector, Kelsey Simons, Colleen Galambos, Robin P. Bonifas, Chris Herman, Deirdre Downes, Jean C. Munn, Giang Rudderham, Elizabeth A. Cordes, and Robert Connolly

2   Serious Mental Illness in Nursing Homes: Roles and Perceived Competence of Social Services Directors   25
Denise Gammonley, Xiaochuan Wang, Kelsey Simons, Kevin M. Smith, and Mercedes Bern-Klug

3   Social Services Involvement in Care Transitions and Admissions in Nursing Homes   44
Colleen Galambos, Laura Rollin, Mercedes Bern-Klug, Mike Oie, and Eric Engelbart

4   Dementia Tops Training Needs of Nursing Home Social Services Directors; Discharge Responsibilities Are Common Core Functions of the Department   62
Mercedes Bern-Klug and Elizabeth Cordes

5   Structural Characteristics of Nursing Homes and Social Service Directors that Influence Their Engagement in Disaster Preparedness Processes   79
Nancy Kusmaul, Susanny Beltran, Tommy Buckley, Allison Gibson, and Mercedes Bern-Klug

6   Social Service Directors' Roles and Self-Efficacy in Suicide Risk Management in US Nursing Homes   95
Xiaochuan Wang, Kelsey Simons, Denise Gammonley, Amy Restorick Roberts, and Mercedes Bern-Klug

7   More Evidence that Federal Regulations Perpetuate Unrealistic Nursing Home
    Social Services Staffing Ratios   115
    Mercedes Bern-Klug, Kara A. Carter, and Yi Wang

8   Barriers to Psychosocial Care in Nursing Homes as Reported by
    Social Services Directors   136
    Amy Restorick Roberts, Kevin Smith, Mercedes Bern-Klug, and Paige Hector

9   Dementia Care Involvement and Training Needs of Social Services Directors in
    U.S. Nursing Homes   155
    Jung Kwak, Kevin M. Smith, Mercedes Bern-Klug, and Kristin Kalin

    Index   167

Citation Information

The chapters in this book were originally published in the *Journal of Gerontological Social Work*, volume 64, issue 7 (2021). When citing this material, please use the original page numbering for each article, as follows:

Introduction
Introducing the Special Issue on Nursing Home Social Services Research
Robin P. Bonifas
Journal of Gerontological Social Work, volume 64, issue 7 (2021) pp. 697–698

Chapter 1
About a Third of Nursing Home Social Services Directors Have Earned a Social Work Degree and License
Mercedes Bern-Klug, Kevin M. Smith, Amy Restorick Roberts, Nancy Kusmaul, Denise Gammonley, Paige Hector, Kelsey Simons, Colleen Galambos, Robin P. Bonifas, Chris Herman, Deirdre Downes, Jean C. Munn, Giang Rudderham, Elizabeth A. Cordes and Robert Connolly
Journal of Gerontological Social Work, volume 64, issue 7 (2021) pp. 699–720

Chapter 2
Serious Mental Illness in Nursing Homes: Roles and Perceived Competence of Social Services Directors
Denise Gammonley, Xiaochuan Wang, Kelsey Simons, Kevin M. Smith and Mercedes Bern-Klug
Journal of Gerontological Social Work, volume 64, issue 7 (2021) pp. 721–739

Chapter 3
Social Services Involvement in Care Transitions and Admissions in Nursing Homes
Colleen Galambos, Laura Rollin, Mercedes Bern-Klug, Mike Oie and Eric Engelbart
Journal of Gerontological Social Work, volume 64, issue 7 (2021) pp. 740–757

Chapter 4
Dementia Tops Training Needs of Nursing Home Social Services Directors; Discharge Responsibilities Are Common Core Functions of the Department
Mercedes Bern-Klug and Elizabeth Cordes
Journal of Gerontological Social Work, volume 64, issue 7 (2021) pp. 758–774

Chapter 5
Structural Characteristics of Nursing Homes and Social Service Directors that Influence Their Engagement in Disaster Preparedness Processes
Nancy Kusmaul, Susanny Beltran, Tommy Buckley, Allison Gibson and Mercedes Bern-Klug
Journal of Gerontological Social Work, volume 64, issue 7 (2021) pp. 775–790

Chapter 6
Social Service Directors' Roles and Self-Efficacy in Suicide Risk Management in US Nursing Homes
Xiaochuan Wang, Kelsey Simons, Denise Gammonley, Amy Restorick Roberts and Mercedes Bern-Klug
Journal of Gerontological Social Work, volume 64, issue 7 (2021) pp. 791–810

Chapter 7
More Evidence that Federal Regulations Perpetuate Unrealistic Nursing Home Social Services Staffing Ratios
Mercedes Bern-Klug, Kara A. Carter and Yi Wang
Journal of Gerontological Social Work, volume 64, issue 7 (2021) pp. 811–831

Chapter 8
Barriers to Psychosocial Care in Nursing Homes as Reported by Social Services Directors
Amy Restorick Roberts, Kevin Smith, Mercedes Bern-Klug and Paige Hector
Journal of Gerontological Social Work, volume 64, issue 7 (2021) pp. 832–850

Chapter 9
Dementia Care Involvement and Training Needs of Social Services Directors in U.S. Nursing Homes
Jung Kwak, Kevin M. Smith, Mercedes Bern-Klug & Kristin Kalin
Journal of Gerontological Social Work, volume 64, issue 7 (2021) pp. 851–862

For any permission-related enquiries please visit:
http://www.tandfonline.com/page/help/permissions

Notes on Contributors

Susanny Beltran, School of Social Work, University of Central Florida, Orlando, USA.

Mercedes Bern-Klug, School of Social Work, University of Iowa, USA.

Robin P. Bonifas, Department of Social Work, John A. Hartford Faculty Scholar in Geriatric Social Work, College of Health and Human Services, Indiana State University, Terre Haute, USA.

Tommy Buckley, School of Social Work, Virginia Commonwealth University, Richmond, USA.

Kara A. Carter, School of Social Work, University of Iowa, USA.

Robert Connolly, Retired CMS Health Insurance Analyst, Marriottsville, USA.

Elizabeth A. Cordes, Social Worker, Maple Manor Village, Aplington, USA.

Deirdre Downes, Social Work and Supportive Care Programs, Isabella Geriatric Center, MJHS, USA.

Eric Engelbart, Milwaukee Center for Independence, USA.

Colleen Galambos, Helen Bader Endowed Chair in Applied Gerontology and Professor, Helen Bader School of Social Welfare, University of Wisconsin Milwaukee, USA.

Denise Gammonley, College of Health Professions and Sciences, Academic Health Sciences Center, University of Central Florida, Orlando, USA.

Allison Gibson, College of Social Work, University of Kentucky, Lexington, USA.

Paige Hector, Paige Ahead Healthcare Education & Consulting, LLC, Tucson, USA.

Chris Herman, Senior Practice Associate–Aging and IRB Chair, National Association of Social Workers (NASW), Washington, USA.

Kristin Kalin, School of Social Work, University of Iowa, USA.

Nancy Kusmaul, Department of Social Work, University of Maryland, Baltimore, USA.

Jung Kwak, School of Nursing, The University of Texas at Austin, USA.

Jean C. Munn, College of Social Work, Florida State University, Tallahassee, USA.

Mike Oie, Social Science Research Center, University of Iowa, USA.

Amy Restorick Roberts, Department of Family Science & Social Work, College of Education, Health & Society, Miami University, Oxford, USA.

Laura Rollin, Helen Bader School of Social Welfare, University of Wisconsin-Milwaukee, USA.

Giang Rudderham, Science Consultant, Iowa Social Science Research Center, University of Iowa, USA.

Kevin M. Smith, Department of Psychological & Quantitative Foundations, University of Iowa, USA.

Kelsey Simons, Department of Psychiatry, VISN 2 Center of Excellence for Suicide Prevention, VA Finger Lakes Health Care System, University of Rochester Medical Center, USA.

Xiaochuan Wang, School of Social Work, College of Health Professions and Sciences, University of Central Florida, Orlando, USA.

Yi Wang, School of Social Work, University of Iowa, USA.

Preface

Home is where you are known, comfortable, safe, and feel a sense of control

Social workers play an important role in helping residents and families feel more "at home" in the nursing home. For most people, in part because it is a group setting, the nursing home will never match the comfort of one's home, yet we could be doing better. When social workers and other staff members have the time, skill, and desire to attend to the emotional and psychosocial aspects of nursing home living and dying, the resident and family experience can be improved. Fellow staff benefit also. The pages that follow highlight various aspects of the social work role and can support the reader in understanding some of the many ways social work services can enhance the nursing home experience.

The terms "social services" and "social work" are used throughout the book. In general, the department is called the social services department. The people who work in that department are either social workers (people with an undergraduate or graduate degree from a Council on Social Work Education [CSWE] accredited social work program) or social services staff (people who may have a college degree, but not in social work). Federal regulations require only nursing homes with more than 120 beds to hire one full-time person in social services. That person, although called a social worker in the federal regulations, is currently not required to have a social work education. Calling people without a social work degree social workers is at odds with the qualifications of social workers in all other health care settings that receive Medicare and/ or Medicaid financial support, as well as out-of-line with the definition of social work held by the National Association of Social Workers and state-licensing boards. Two-thirds of the nursing homes in the US have fewer than 120 beds, and therefore are not required by federal law to hire even one person in social services, although our data reveal that many do (see chapter 1). A well-prepared and highly motivated social worker is necessary for excellent psychosocial care in the nursing home setting, but those qualities are not sufficient to guarantee excellent psychosocial care. A reasonable ratio of residents per social worker is also needed (see chapter 7).

This collection of articles would not have been possible without the financial support of the RRF Foundation for Aging. This foundation has a long and stellar history of providing funds to people seeking to improve the experience of older adulthood, including but not limited to persons in nursing homes. The RRF Foundation for Aging supported online and paper and pencil data collection efforts. They also supported preliminary data analyses. I would also like to acknowledge and thank members of the study's advisory committee. Not only did they help finetune the survey instrument, many also took on the responsibility of authoring articles using the data. I would like to thank my consultant Dr. Rosalie Kane (RIP) for her leadership, enthusiasm, and insight into nursing home social services and overall resident quality of life. She made significant contributions to the knowledge base during her decades of scholarship in the area of long-term services and supports. She died in 2020—during the pandemic and during the time when the data collected for this study were being analyzed. The project benefited from her expertise in 2018 and 2019 when the study was being planned and the data collected. I'd also like to thank the readers who will take this information and run with it, all the way "home" to a better nursing home experience for residents, family, and staff.

Mercedes Bern-Klug, PhD, MSW, MA
Professor, School of Social Work
University of Iowa
John A. Hartford Geriatric Social Work Faculty Scholar

Introduction: Nursing Home Social Services Research

Robin P. Bonifas

Dear Readers,

I am pleased to introduce this special issue that features research from the 2019 National Nursing Home Social Services Directors Study. I am so proud of my colleagues' work in this area! Funded by the Retirement Research Foundation, this survey study involved a national sample of 924 directors of social services departments in nursing homes certified to receive Medicare and/or Medicaid funds. Data were gathered about the barriers to resident care provision, the structure and role of the social services department, the training needs of social services personnel, and their employment benefits, compensation, and job satisfaction.

The manuscripts in this issue address a range of issues salient to nursing home social workers and nursing home social work practices: realistic staffing ratios, qualification levels, dementia training needs, involvement in care transitions and admissions, barriers to psychosocial care, and roles in addressing specific resident needs: serious mental health, suicide risk, and disaster preparedness. Be sure to experience a new feature of the *Journal of Gerontological Social Work*: brief video introductions by the authors of some of these papers available at:

https://youtu.be/emZNvlQ372M

About one-third of nursing home social services directors have earned a social work degree and license.

https://youtu.be/nodB_y82X3Q

More evidence that federal regulations perpetuate unrealistic nursing home social services staffing ratios.

https://youtu.be/Ckko45vHoXo

Dementia tops training needs of nursing home social services directors. Discharge . . . .

Readers may notice I am an author on one of the manuscripts in this issue and wonder about procedures for managing the dual roles of being an author and editor-in-chief. The strategy to address this potentially problematic situation is that I am blinded to the entire review process for my own manuscripts; all procedures are managed by the associate editor, Dr. Megumi Inoue, who serves as the editor-in-chief in my stead. The following story will illustrate the level of blinding I experienced for my own papers . . .

In my role as editor-in-chief, Dr. Bern-Klug contacted me to check on the status of the "About a third of nursing home social services . . . " paper. Forgetting I was an author on that one, I used the paper's identification number to search the manuscript review system, so I could effectively answer her question. I repeatedly received the message "The manuscript does not exist" and started to panic because I thought the manuscript had been lost somewhere in the void. Imagine the horror of losing a colleague's carefully prepared manuscript! Our managing editor, Hwei-Wern Shen, quickly assured me the manuscript was present and accounted for, but I could not see it because I was blinded as an author on the paper. Ha-ha!

Please enjoy this issue's articles based on the 2019 National Nursing Home Social Services Directors Study.

Robin P. Bonifas

About a Third of Nursing Home Social Services Directors Have Earned a Social Work Degree and License

Mercedes Bern-Klug ⓘ, Kevin M. Smith, Amy Restorick Roberts,
Nancy Kusmaul ⓘ, Denise Gammonley , Paige Hector , Kelsey Simons ,
Colleen Galambos, Robin P. Bonifas, Chris Herman, Deirdre Downes,
Jean C. Munn, Giang Rudderham, Elizabeth A. Cordes, and Robert Connolly

ABSTRACT
Nursing home (NH) residents have high psychosocial needs related to illness, disability, and changing life circumstances. The staff member with the most expertise in addressing psychosocial needs is the social worker. However, federal regulations indicate that only NHs with 120+ beds need hire a social services staff member and that a "qualified social worker" need not have a social work degree. Therefore, two-thirds of NHs are not required to employ a social services staff member and none are required to hire a degreed social worker. This is in stark contrast to NASW professional standards. Reporting findings from this nationally representative sample of 924 social services directors, we describe the NH social services workforce and document that most NHs do hire social services staff, although 42% of social services directors are not social work educated. 37% of NHs have a degreed and licensed social worker at the helm of social services. The odds of hiring a degreed and licensed social workers are higher for larger NHs, especially if not-for-profit and not part of a chain. NH residents deserve psychosocial care planned by staff with such expertise. Quality of psychosocial care impacts quality of life.

Nursing home residents have serious health concerns. The federal government reports that about half of residents are living with dementia, 26% with arthritis, 46% with depression, 38% with heart disease, 32% with diabetes, and 71% with hypertension (Harris-Kojetin et al., 2019, p. 22). Many residents are dealing with grief and loss (Drageset et al., 2015). Some residents, including some with dementia, have behaviors that are troublesome to other residents (e.g., kicking, biting, yelling) that can sometimes be effectively addressed using nonpharmacological approaches (Bonifas, 2016), if trained staff are available. This constellation of needs is ripe for the development or exacerbation of psychosocial needs among nursing home residents. The skills to identify and address these psychosocial needs are in the social work wheelhouse. Despite the widespread recognition of the prevalence of psychosocial issues, there has been little national attention on the staff member most prepared to anticipate and address resident psychosocial issues, the social worker. While all staff are responsible for identifying these concerns and the interdisciplinary team should be developing care plans to address psychosocial issues, psychosocial issues are a central aspect of the social work role.

Nursing home social services departments (which may include professional social workers who hold a social work degree and license and/or para-professional social services staff) identify and address resident emotional and psychosocial needs and provide support to residents' family members (however the resident defines family). They not only assist with transitions to, within, and from nursing homes, they also support residents and families in coping with interpersonal challenges and making health-related decisions. In so doing, social services staff contribute in fundamental ways to day-to-day nursing home operations, including assisting in maintaining the daily census. Nursing home social services staff members are typically charged with ensuring staff, residents, and family members understand and honor residents' rights. They respond to resident and family grievances and build on their strengths. These important tasks and processes directly impact residents' quality of life. Yet, little is known about the characteristics of staff who are employed in nursing home social services departments. In this paper, we refer to the department as social services and to the employee as either a social services staff member or if the employee has an undergraduate or graduate degree in social work, as a social worker.

The purpose of this article is to report characteristics of the social services department with special attention paid to the characteristics of the director of social services; compare these characteristics with data collected in 2006; and identify characteristics of nursing homes most likely to employ a degreed (baccalaureate or master's degree in social work) and licensed social worker as the director of social services.

Background

This section describes qualification expectations for nursing home social services staff held by government and the social work profession. After describing state licensure of social workers in general, we compare and contrast two definitions of qualified social workers in the nursing home context, the National Association of Social Workers' (NASW) definition and that of the federal government, and then conclude by speaking to the variation in state qualifications of social services staff in the context of nursing homes.

State licensure of social workers

In the U.S., the licensing of professionals, including social workers, occurs at the state level. The Association of Social Work Boards (ASWB) is a nonprofit association that collects and disseminates social work regulations in the U.S. and Canada. The ASWB website reports that as of July 2020, all 50 states and the District of Columbia license the practice of social work at the master's level (MSW) and most (41) also license at the bachelor's level (BSW) (Association of Social Work Boards, 2018). Data also indicate that most (46) jurisdictions have both social work practice and title protections and that the remaining five have either title or practice protection. "In jurisdictions with title protection and/or practice act protection, only licensed social workers are qualified or permitted to call themselves social workers and practice the profession" (Association of Social Work Boards, 2018).

Although all states and the District of Columbia license the practice of social work and have either title or practice protection, 37 states have exemptions that allow nonsocial workers to engage in social work practice, in specific circumstances related to the individual (for example, being grandfathered into the role), or by setting. Twenty-two states have exemptions that allow non-social workers to act as social workers in state government settings, 18 in federal government settings, three states exempt assisted living, and two states (Louisiana and North Dakota) exempt "social work designees" in skilled nursing facilities provided they work under the direction of a licensed social worker (Association of Social Work Boards, 2018). The Florida statute detailing the practice of social work clarifies that title protection does not extend to "employees providing social work services under administrative supervision in long-term care facilities licensed by the Agency for Health Care Administration" (Florida Statutes, 2020, section 491.016). Therefore, despite title protection, in many nursing homes throughout the country, state laws allow exceptions for the title of "social worker" to be used by people who have otherwise not met minimum state requirements.

Table 1. Definitions of a qualified social worker in the nursing home setting.

NASW	CMS
A social worker has, at minimum, a bachelor's degree from an accredited school or program of social work; has two years of post-graduate experience in long-term care or related programs; and meets equivalent state requirements for social work practice . . . . In no instance should a social worker have less than a baccalaureate degree from an accredited school of program of social work. (NASW, 2003, page, p. 7) The NASW standards also address the qualifications of the director of social services in a nursing home: The term *social work director* is defined in these standards as a social worker who is the staff member responsible for the social work program in the facility. It is preferable that the social work director be a graduate of a master's degree program from an accredited school or program of social work, have a minimum of two years post-graduate experience in long-term care or related programs, and meet equivalent state requirements for social work practice . . . .(NASW, 2003, page, p. 8)	(1) An individual with a minimum of a bachelor's degree in social work or a bachelor's degree in a human services field including, but not limited to, sociology, gerontology, special education, rehabilitation counseling, and psychology; and (2) One year of supervised social work experience in a health care setting working directly with individuals. (CFR, §483.70, Code of Federal Regulations, 2020). Director of social services: no definition

Professional standards for nursing home social workers

As reported in Table 1 professional standards for social work practice in long-term care facilities set by the National Association of Social Workers (NASW), the largest professional social work organization in the U.S., require at a minimum a bachelor's degree in social work and recommend a social worker with a master's degree for the position of social services director (NASW, 2003). Nursing homes social workers are expected to meet state requirements for social work practice and to have post-graduate experience in long-term care settings. The NASW qualifications are in significant contrast to those put forth by the Centers for Medicare and Medicaid Services (CMS), the federal agency responsible for nursing home regulations.

Federal government rules for nursing home social workers

CMS requires the nation's 15,578 nursing homes to comply with federal, state, and local laws in order to obtain and maintain certification in the Medicare and/or Medicaid programs (CFR, §483.70, Code of Federal Regulations, 2020). Furthermore, the Code of Federal Regulations (CFR) states that the services provided or arranged by the facility for residents, must-

    (i) Meet professional standards of quality.
  (ii) Be provided by qualified persons in accordance with each resident's written plan of care.
 (iii) Be culturally competent and trauma informed (CFR, §483.21, Code of Federal Regulations, 2020).

In addition, the CFR has this requirement of all certified nursing homes: "(1) The facility must employ on a full-time, part-time or consultant basis those professionals necessary to carry out the provisions of these requirements. (2) Professional staff must be licensed, certified, or registered in accordance with applicable State laws" (CFR, §483.70, Code of Federal Regulations, 2020).

Federal regulations also require that Medicare and/or Medicaid certified nursing homes provide care to help residents remain healthy and maintain function as long as possible. The requirements for care go beyond physical care to encompass psychosocial care that promotes resident dignity, self-determination, social interaction, and engagement in meaningful activities (CMS, State Operations Manual, CMS, 2017). The CFR states, "the facility must provide medically-related social services to attain or maintain the highest practicable physical, mental and psychosocial well-being of each resident" (CFR, §483.40, Code of Federal Regulations, 2020). The quality of psychosocial care delivered in nursing homes has been linked with both the presence of social service staff and with facility characteristics, "psychosocial care quality was better in facilities where State requirements for qualified social services staffing exceeded federal minimum regulations . . . For-profit status and higher percentage of Medicaid residents are associated with lower quality (Zhang et al., 2008, p. 5). In addition, Roberts et al. (2019) report that resident outcomes (including reduction of behavioral symptoms and ability to return home after receiving post-acute care) are associated with higher qualifications of social services staff.

Although all certified nursing homes are required to meet residents' psychosocial needs, facilities can do so in one of two ways. If a nursing home has 120 or fewer beds, CMS allows the facility to contract with a local agency or individual to provide medically related psychosocial services to residents. If a nursing home has more than 120 beds, it is required to employ one full-time "qualified social worker." This requirement is problematic on three accounts. First, most (70%) of the nation's 15,578 certified nursing homes have fewer than 120 beds (see Table 3) consequently this requirement does not apply to them; second, the federal operationalization of "qualified social worker" in a nursing home does not meet professional standards and is at odds with other federal definitions of "qualified social worker" in other Medicare and Medicaid certified settings because it does not require a social work license and a degree from an accredited social work program; and third, the "120 bed" rule is arbitrary (Bern-Klug, 2018, supplemental materials) and runs counter to evidence from nationally representative samples of nursing home social services directors, a majority of whom reported that one full-time social worker could meet the psychosocial needs of 60 *or fewer* long-term care residents (and an even smaller case load of post-acute residents) (Bern-Klug et al., 2021, 2010).

The federal rules for nursing homes to participate in Medicare and Medicaid were updated in 2016. During the public comment period, a number of groups requested that the rules for social services be strengthened by setting social services staffing ratios that reflect the growth in proportion of nursing home post-acute/skilled residents and by requiring all "qualified social workers" to have a baccalaureate or master's degree in social work. CMS disagreed. Not only did CMS decide against requiring a social work education to be considered a qualified social worker in a nursing home, but they also added a new "human services" degree option: "Thus we are finalizing the social worker qualifications as section 483.70(p) as proposed, with 'gerontology' as an example of a human services field that an individual with a bachelor's degree could qualify as a social worker in a LTC facility" (Federal Register, 2016, page 68801). It is unclear how CMS decides which degrees qualify as "human services" and on what basis a "human services-related degree" is equivalent to a social work degree, especially given that some of the CMS-listed "human services" undergraduate degrees, such as sociology, psychology, and gerontology do not require an internship or direct practice at the individual and organizational levels, and do not require coursework that teaches practice skills relevant to assessing and addressing psychosocial issues such as: crisis intervention, counseling, psychosocial assessment, psychosocial care planning, person-centered advocacy, screening for abuse, suicide risk assessment, group processes, and engaging in difficult conversations. A social work education does.

State regulations regarding nursing home social services

Although the federal government has lax personnel qualifications for nursing home social workers that are in direct opposition to long standing professional standards, each state has the option of following the federal rules or developing more stringent rules, which might be a better fit to their own state laws related to the practice of social work. For the most part, state nursing home rules related to social work qualifications are also lax as well as in opposition to professional standards, and in some cases counter to their own state laws pertaining to the licensing of the practice of social work. A 2018 review of all administrative codes (Bern-Klug et al, 2018) for the 50 states and the District of Columbia reports that 12 states do not address nursing home social work qualifications, 25 states appear to be out of compliance with federal rules, and only one state – Maine–appears to meet the NASW standards.

The objectives of this study were to: 1) describe the current characteristics of the nation's social services directors and departments; 2) compare 2019 characteristics with 2006 characteristics; and 3) identify nursing home characteristics associated with employing a degreed and licensed social worker as social services director. A similar study was undertaken in 2006 (Bern-Klug et al., 2009).

Methods

In January 2019, a simple random sample of 3,650 of the 15,578 Medicare and/ or Medicaid certified nursing homes listed on the December 2018 CMS Nursing Home Compare Database (available to the public at medicare.gov) was drawn using SPSS version 25 using the random sample generator command. For each of the nursing homes in the sample, the mailing address and phone number were downloaded from the CMS Nursing Home Compare database, along with selected other data, such as whether the facility was Medicare and/or Medicaid certified, tax status, and ownership. Additional variables, such as whether the nursing home was part of a chain, were downloaded from the CMS Provider of Service (POS) database, also publicly available online.

Participants

For this study, the target respondent was the director of social services. During spring 2019, students and staff at the University of Iowa's Iowa Social Science Research Center telephoned each of the 3,650 nursing homes in the sample to determine eligibility for the study, i.e., whether at least one social services staff person was employed at least part-time. For each eligible nursing home, callers asked for the social services director's name and e-mail and verified the nursing home's postal address. Phone calls documented that the vast majority (84%) of the 3,067 (of the 3,650) nursing homes employed at least one social services staff person (full or part-time) at the time of the phone call. If the nursing home did not employ social services staff, the nursing home was dropped from the sample. Other reasons for exclusion from the study include: the nursing home was in the process of hiring social services staff, the social services staff member was on leave, the phone number was disconnected or incorrect, the phone was not answered (we let the phone ring 10 times on three different days/times), or the call went directly to an answering machine.

If an e-mail address for the social services director was secured, an invitation to participate in the study was emailed. In addition to including each potential respondent's first and last name, the subject line also read: *Because you are an expert*. The e-mail message addressed the potential respondent by first and last name, explained the purpose of the study, and provided a link to the online Qualtrics survey. If there was no response to the e-mail invitation and follow-up (or if callers were not successful in securing the e-mail address of the social services director during the screening phone call), a hard copy of the questionnaire was mailed to the nursing home social services director. Efforts to improve the postal mail response rate included mailing the questionnaire in a bright green oversize envelop, placing a combination of six colorful postage stamps (by hand) on each envelop, including a magnet in the mailing that read, "*Because you are an expert … .*". and addressing the potential respondent by their first and last name. Respondents were not compensated for participation. The study procedures were approved by the University of Iowa's Human Subjects Office and funded by the RRF Foundation for Aging. Of the 3,067nursing home social services directors invited to participate, 924 completed the survey (536 online and 388 on paper), for a response rate of 30%.

Instrument

A similar study was undertaken in 2006 and that survey instrument served as the basis for the 2019 study. A group of 13 national advisors (among the coauthors) with experience in nursing home research and/or nursing home social services practice met online four times to discuss the survey methods and questions. The questionnaire was extensively reviewed by these advisors and pilot tested with five current nursing home social services directors who discussed the questionnaire with the principal investigator after completing it.

The questionnaire consisted of 185 items including six open-ended questions. Sections of the survey used the same question stem to reduce respondent burden. Social services directors were asked to report the extent to which the social services department was involved in 46 tasks, inspired by the NASW's and the Veteran's Health Administration's descriptions of nursing home social services responsibilities, as summarized in Simons et al. (2012). Questions addressed barriers to providing social and emotional care, training needs, departmental staffing, job satisfaction, and compensation. Online respondents took on average 45 minutes to complete the questionnaire (no similar data are available regarding completion time for paper respondents). Completed and returned paper questionnaires were double entered.

Measures

The study's database contains data from three sources: two CMS public datafiles and the data provided by respondents. To reduce respondent burden, data describing the nursing home that could be easily secured from public access datafiles on the CMS website were downloaded and added to the respondent data. The following data were downloaded from the Nursing Home Compare website (https://data.medicare.gov/data/nursing-home-compare):

Beds
Number of Medicare and/or Medicaid certified beds.

Ownership
CMS's 13 categories of tax status were collapsed into three for this study: for profit, not-for-profit, and government.

Type of facility
There were four possible values based on whether the facility was Medicare certified as a skilled nursing facility (SNF) or Medicaid certified as a nursing facility (NF), or dually certified in Medicare and Medicaid, or considered a "distinct part" of a larger system or institution and fiscally separate.

CMS quality rating
These data were developed from resident assessments and Medicare claims data and reflect clinical measures such as weight loss, flu shot administration, number of resident falls resulting in major injury. The quality rating data were combined with two other components (staffing data for registered nurses (RNs) and licensed practical nurses (LPNs) and health inspection results) to determine the nursing home's "star rating" which is publicly available online (https://www.medicare.gov/nursinghomecompare/search.html?). Due to concerns about the reliability of the staffing data, only the quality rating data were used in this study.

Census regions and divisions
The CMS database contained the street address of each certified nursing home. For this study state information was used to categorize nursing homes into the four census regions which are further divided into nine census divisions (https://www2.census.gov/geo/pdfs/maps-data/maps/reference/us_regdiv.pdf). The Midwest West division is the reference category for the logistic regression analysis.

RUCC
County data were used to categorize nursing homes into one of nine Rural Urban Continuum Codes (RUCC). Counties were classified by population size and for non-metropolitan counties whether the county was adjacent to a metropolitan county. The RUCC were developed in 2013 by the USDA (https://www.ers.usda.gov/data-products/rural-urban-continuum-codes.aspx). The July 2019 RUCC county designation was used in this study. In the logistic regression analysis, the reference category for RUCC was non-metropolitan counties with a population of 20,000 or more and adjacent to a metro county.

Metro/nonmetro

The nine RUCC were collapsed into a dichotomous variable metro or non-metro counties.

Chain

In addition to data downloaded from the CMS Nursing Home Compare website listed above, data indicating whether each nursing home was part of a chain of two or more facilities was downloaded from the CMS Provider of Services datafile (https://www.cms.gov/Research-Statistics-Data-and-Systems/Downloadable-Public-Use-Files/Provider-of-Services) and added to the study database.

Eleven hard copies of the questionnaire were completed and returned without a useable study ID number because the respondent removed the ID number, or an incorrect ID number was written on the questionnaire. Consequently, the respondent data on those 11 completed surveys could not be linked with CMS facility characteristics data.

Analyses

Descriptive statistics were used to compare the sample characteristics with population characteristics of 15,578 nursing homes. Frequencies were used to

Table 2. Geographic comparison of sample to population of U.S. certified nursing homes: 2019.

	Population*	Sample
	N = 15,578	n = 911
County Classification – Office of Management and Budget		
Metropolitan	72%	67%
Non Metropolitan	28	33
Rural Urban Continuum Code (USDA) County Classification		
1 Metro 1 million +	41	33
2 Metro 250,000–1 million	20	20
3 Metro <250,000	11	13
4 Nonmetro 20,000+ urban, adjacent to metro	6	6
5 Nonmetro 20,000+ urban, not adjacent to metro	3	3
6 Nonmetro 2,500–19,999 urban, adjacent to metro	9	9
7 Nonmetro 2,500–19,000 urban, not adjacent to metro	6	7
8 Nonmetro completely rural or <2,500 urban, adjacent to metro	2	3
9 Nonmetro completely rural or <2,500 urban and not adjacent to metro	3	5
Census Bureau's 4 Regions		
Northeast	17	16
Midwest	33	41
South	35	29
West	16	14
Census Bureau's 9 Divisions		
1 Northeast: New England	6	7
2 Northeast: Mid-Atlantic	11	9
3 Midwest: East North Central	20	21
4 Midwest: West North Central	13	21
5 South: South Atlantic	15	14
6 South: East South Central	7	6
7 South: West South Central	13	10
8 West: Mountain	5	6
9 West: Pacific	10	7

*National data are from the December 2018 CMS Nursing Home Compare dataset.

compare survey data from the previous 2006 sample and the current 2019 sample. Logistic regression was used to estimate the likelihood that a nursing home employs a licensed and degreed social worker as the director of social services. SPSS version 26 was used for the analyses along with the Hayes PROCESS MACRO V 3.3, Model 3 for multiple moderation analyses that were part of building the logistic regression model (Hayes, 2017).

Results

Nursing home facility characteristics

As shown in Table 2, the geographic characteristics of nursing homes in the sample were similar to the national population of Medicare and/or Medicaid certified nursing homes, with most of the differences within five percent. Most of the nation's nursing homes were in metropolitan counties which were slightly underrepresented in the sample (72% of the population and 67% of the sample). Of the four census regions represented in Table 2, the Midwest region was slightly over-represented. Nursing home characteristics were similar between the online and paper respondents.

Table 3 compares the sample to the population of nursing homes in terms of the type of facility, ownership/tax status, number of beds, and chain status. The percentages of different types of facilities in the sample mirrored the national population of nursing homes, although for-profit facilities were slightly underrepresented. The majority of nursing homes in the sample and

Table 3. Comparison of nursing home characteristics: sample to population of U.S. certified nursing homes: 2019.

	Population* N = 15,578	Sample, n = 911
Type of facility		
SNF/NF (dual)	78	79
SNF/NF (distinct part)	15	16
SNF	5	2
NF	2	3
Tax status/ownership		
For Profit	70	63
Not-for-Profit	23	29
Government	7	8
Number of beds		
Less than 60	19	20
61–120	52	53
121 or more	29	27
Part of a chain of 2 or more nursing homes	59	58
CMS quality rating		
1-Much below average	5	5
2-Below average	10	10
3-Average	14	16
4-Above average	22	22
5-Much above average	49	48

National data are from December 2018 CMS Nursing Home Care dataset, with the exception of "chain status" which is from the CMS Provider of Services dataset.

Table 4. Comparison of characteristics of nursing home social services directors: 2006 and 2019.

	2006 Sample	2019 Sample
	n = 1,071	*n* = 924
Women	93%	92%
Race		
African American	6	6
White	90	88
Age-group		
18–25	5	4
26–34	23	24
35–44	25	24
45–54	29	23
55–64	15	19
65+	2	5
Highest Education		
High School	14	10
Associates Degree	6	6
Bachelors (non-SW)	24	20
Bachelors (SW)	31	30
Masters (non-SW)	8	7
Masters (SW)	17	28
SW Licensed or Certified	39	47
Annual Salary for		
Full-time Staff		
<$30,000	25	8
$30k – 39,999	42	20
$40k – 49,999	22	26
$50k – 59,999	8	25
$60,000 or more	3	20
Years of NH Social Services Experience		
Less than 1	7	7
1–3 years	20	19
4–9 years	34	27
10–15 years	18	16
More than 15 years	21	31
Plans to work in a NH in two years	81	81

in the country were dually certified to accept both Medicare and Medicaid. Table 3 also shows the sample was representative of the population in terms of CMS quality ratings.

Social services directors' characteristics

Table 4 compares characteristics of nursing home social services directors in 2019 with values from the 2006 sample. In both years, women constituted

Table 5. Percent of nursing home social services directors who report holding a social work license/certification, by highest educational attainment: 2019.

Education	Percent of sample	Percent reporting a social work license or certification
Less than 4-year degree	16%	31%
Bachelors (non-SW)	20	19
Bachelors (SW)	30	54
Masters (non-SW)	7	33
Masters (SW)	29	72
	100%	47%
With BSW or MSW	59%	63%

more than 90% of social services directors, and most directors reported their race as white. A small percentage of respondents reported their age as 25 or younger (5% in 2006 and 4% in 2019). In 2006, 17% of the respondents were age 55 or older and that percentage increased to 24% in the 2019 sample, evidence of the aging of the social services director work force. The percentage of social services directors with a social work degree increased from 48% in 2006 to 59% in 2019. A higher percentage of the 2019 sample (28%) had earned a master's degree in social work compare to the 2006 sample (17%). The percentage of respondents who were social work licensed or certified increased from 39% in 2006 to 47% in 2019. Table 4 shows that salaries for full-time staff increased over the 13-year period between studies, with the percentage reporting earnings of 50,000 USD or more per year increasing from 11% in 2006 to 45% in 2019 (the salaries are listed as reported by respondents, they were not adjusted for inflation).

Table 5 provides a summary of the educational attainment of the social services directors and the percentage of each educational category who reported having a state-issued social work license or certification. Over half of the BSW respondents and almost three-fourths (72%) of MSW respondents had earned a state-issued social work license or certification. In all, about two-thirds (63%) of directors with a social work degree (BSW or MSW) were licensed in social work. Reflecting state laws allowing nonsocial workers to obtain a social work license or certification, about one-third of respondents without a social work degree reported having obtained a state-issued social work license or certification.

Additional information (not shown in tables) about the 2019 sample indicated that about half (54%) of social services departments had only one staff person, 31% had two staff members, and 9% had three staff members. Six percent of nursing homes in the sample had four or more people working in the social services department (full or part-time). The vast majority of social services director respondents (93%) were employed full-time (35 hours or more per week), with five percent employed for 20–34 hours per week. Most (80%) reported they expect to be working in nursing homes in two years. More than half (56%) reported they were sometimes "on-call" during evenings and weekends. Also, 61% indicated they "strongly agreed" with the statement asking if they enjoyed working in nursing home social services. In terms of experience level, in both 2006 and 2019, seven percent of the sample reported having less than a year of nursing home social work experience. The percent with 15 or more years of experience increased from 21% in the 2006 sample to 31% in the 2019 sample.

Respondents were asked about a reasonable staffing ratio. Two-thirds of respondents said one full-time social services staff person could assess and care-plan for the psychosocial needs of 59 or fewer residents receiving long-term care and 53% reported that one full-time social worker could address

Table 6. Logistic regression model predicting nursing homes hiring licensed & degreed social workers.

	UOR	95% CI	AOR	95% CI
Step 1	-		$\chi^2(4) = 30.29; p < .001$	
Beds (ref 60–120 beds)				
Less than 60	-	-	0.37***	[.240, .564]
60 to 120	-	-	0.58**	[.421, .795]
Chain Status	-	-	0.99	[.736, 1.332]
Ownership/Tax status	-	-	1.67**	[1.228, 2.280]
Step 2	-		$\chi^2(20) = 119.30; p < .001$	
Bed Size				
Less than 60	0.44***	[.288, .657]	0.58*	[.350, .947]
60 to 120	0.58**	[.422, .793]	0.70*	[.495, .998]
Chain Status	1.15	[.872, 1.511]	0.91	[.660, 1.240]
Ownership	1.46**	[1.101, 1.923]	1.76**	[1.257, 2.454]
RUCC County				
M 1 million plus	1.56	[.844, 2.874]	1.71	[.890, 3.293]
M 250k – 1 million	1.02	[.536, 1.946]	1.06	[.538, 2.105]
M < 250k	1.02	[.516, 2.023]	1.08	[.528, 2.222]
NM 20k plus	0.88	[.331, 2.310]	0.78	[.277, 2.194]
NM 2.5k – 19k adj	0.96	[.462, 1.975]	1.00	[.466, 2.152]
NM 2.5k – 19k	1.10	[.507, 2.374]	1.02	[.453, 2.314]
NM <2.5k adj	0.18*	[.037, 0.837]	0.18*	[.037, .891]
NM <2.5k	0.47	[.188, 1.192]	0.44†	[.163, 1.165]
Census Division				
New England	2.07*	[1.144, 3.731]	1.42	[.749, 2.686]
Mid-Atlantic	1.74*	[1.028, 2.961]	0.96	[.531, 1.745]
Midwest East	1.14	[.740, 1.744]	0.84	[.525, 1.350]
South Atlantic	0.71	[.427, 1.185]	0.51*	[.291, .896]
South East	1.84†	[.979, 3.444]	1.49	[.759, 2.923]
South West	3.44***	[2.029, 5.842]	2.61**	[1.452, 4.677]
West Mountain	0.76	[.388, 1.471]	0.61	[.298, 1.236]
West Pacific	0.17***	[.064, .436]	0.12***	[.043, .311]

UOR = Unadjusted Odds Ratios; AOR = Adjusted Odds Ratios; CI = Confidence Interval; NH = Nursing Home; Chain Status 1 = Chain NH, 2 = Not a Chain NH; Ownership 1 = For Profit NH; 2 = Nonprofit/Government Owned NH; Bed Size reference = 121 or more; RUCC reference = Non Metro county of 20,000+, adjacent to a metro county; Census Division reference = Midwest West division.
$^\dagger p < .1$, *$p < .05$, **$p < .01$, ***$p < .001$.

the needs of 20 or fewer people receiving post-acute care in the nursing homes. Additional information about staffing ratios from this study are available (Bern-Klug et al., 2021).

Logistic regression

A bivariate logistic model was utilized to determine the likelihood of nursing homes employing a licensed and degreed social worker as social services director. Minimal missingness for both regression analyses were identified; a minimal 1.5% of the sample was missing for both the binary logistic regression and the multiple moderation models. Testing variables were examined for collinearity and to determine if any independent variables had a VIF of above 5 (Craney & Surles, 2002); none was noted.

Results for the binary logistic model are provided in Table 6, which is separated into two primary columns. The left column contains unadjusted (i.e., bivariate) odds ratios between the dependent variable and each independent variable. The right column contains adjusted odds ratios where the dependent variable is predicted based on the full logistic model, controlling for the effects of the other independent variables. Overall, model significance was examined for the final step of the full logistic model and a statistically different outcome compared to the null hypothesis ($\chi^2(20)$ = 119.30; $p < .001$) was found. In other words, this set of independent variables contributes beyond chance to predicting which nursing homes employed a degreed and licensed social worker as social services director. The final model's Nagelkerke pseudo-R^2 was 17%. Two variables accounted for 12.5% of the variance: RUCC and census division (discussed below). Finally, it is important to mention that the Odds Ratios (OR) and increases/decreases in likelihood through numbered percentages (%) should be interpreted as increased/decreased chances of correctly predicting whether the nursing home employed a degreed licensed social worker compared to having a 50/50% outcome, which is the assumed null hypothesis. Results in the form of ORs should not be read as a 1:1 ratio or slope-based interpretation.

Compared with non-metropolitan counties with a population of 20,000 or more adjacent to a metro county (the reference group) only the group of non-metropolitan counties with fewer than 2,500 persons and adjacent to a metro county had a statistically different (much lower) odds of employing a licensed and degreed social worker. In fact, with the OR of .18, they were 82% less likely [1 − .18 = .82] to hire a degreed and licensed social worker as social services director.

Compared with nursing homes in the Midwest West region, only nursing homes in the West Pacific census division were less likely to employ a licensed and degreed social worker (OR = 0.17; 83% lesser likelihood; See Table 6). Three divisions were more likely than the Midwest West to employ a licensed and degreed social worker as social services director, with the South West division having the highest likelihood (OR = 3.44; 244% greater likelihood), followed by the New England division (OR = 2.07; 107% greater likelihood) and the Mid-Atlantic (OR = 1.74; 74% greater likelihood). The South East division was trending toward significance (OR = 1.84; 84% greater likelihood) as compared with the Midwest West division, in terms of employing a degreed and licensed social work as social services director.

Adjusted model. Focusing on the full (adjusted for the impact of the other variables in the model) logistic regression model (set of columns on the right of Table 6), the OR of non-metropolitan completely rural counties with less than 2,500 people and adjacent to a metropolitan county remained consistent by being 82% less likely to have a licensed and degreed social worker (OR = 0.18) in both models. For most of the other variables, the unadjusted odds ratios changed when the effect of the other independent variables were accounted for in the adjusted odds ratios.

In the adjusted model, nursing homes in the South West division remained the most likely to employ a degreed and licensed social worker (OR = 2.61; 161% greater likelihood). Two divisions were less likely than the Midwest West to employ a degreed and licensed social worker, South Atlantic (OR = 0.51; 49% less likelihood) and West Pacific (OR = 0.12; 88% less likelihood).

Interaction analyses

Interaction terms were included in the initial logistic models among three variables: bed size groups, ownership types, and chain status of nursing homes, which resulted in three 2-way interaction terms, and one three-way interaction term. The three-way interaction term was found to be significant ($p < .05$) indicating a need to test further moderation effects of those three variables. Therefore, a multiple moderation model was conducted including all independent variables on the same dependent variable (employs a licensed and degreed social worker). Due to the determination of an interaction [moderation effects] among bed size groups, chain status, and ownership type, the values for those three variables as shown in Table 6 should not be interpreted separate from the interaction analysis. Those three variables remain in the initial step of the logistic model to control for their effects on RUCCs and census divisions as well as for consistency of the regression models.

Moderation effects

A multiple moderation model utilizing the dependent variable of a licensed and degreed social worker and the same independent variables as the full logistic model was conducted to determine interactional dynamics among nursing home bed size categories, dichotomous ownership types, and dichotomous chain status. To retain consistency of the analyses, the predictor variables RUCCs and census divisions were included as model covariates, but not in their original form. To prevent the number of predictors in the model from going beyond that recommended for a binary outcome model (Hosmer et al., 2013), the RUCC variable was dummy coded into metro/non-metro counties and the Census divisions variable was effect coded into three dichotomous variables (with the West Pacific region used as the reference group). The full model for multiple moderation was identified to be significant ($\chi^2(15) = 76.22$; $p < .001$) and yielded a Nagelkerke Pseudo-R^2 of 11.1%.

Results indicate several moderation effects by the two moderators (chain status and bed size) and predictor (ownership type) variable on the dependent outcome. The highest order unconditional interaction was determined to be significant ($\chi^2(2) = 6.54$; $p < .05$). To interpret at which levels the

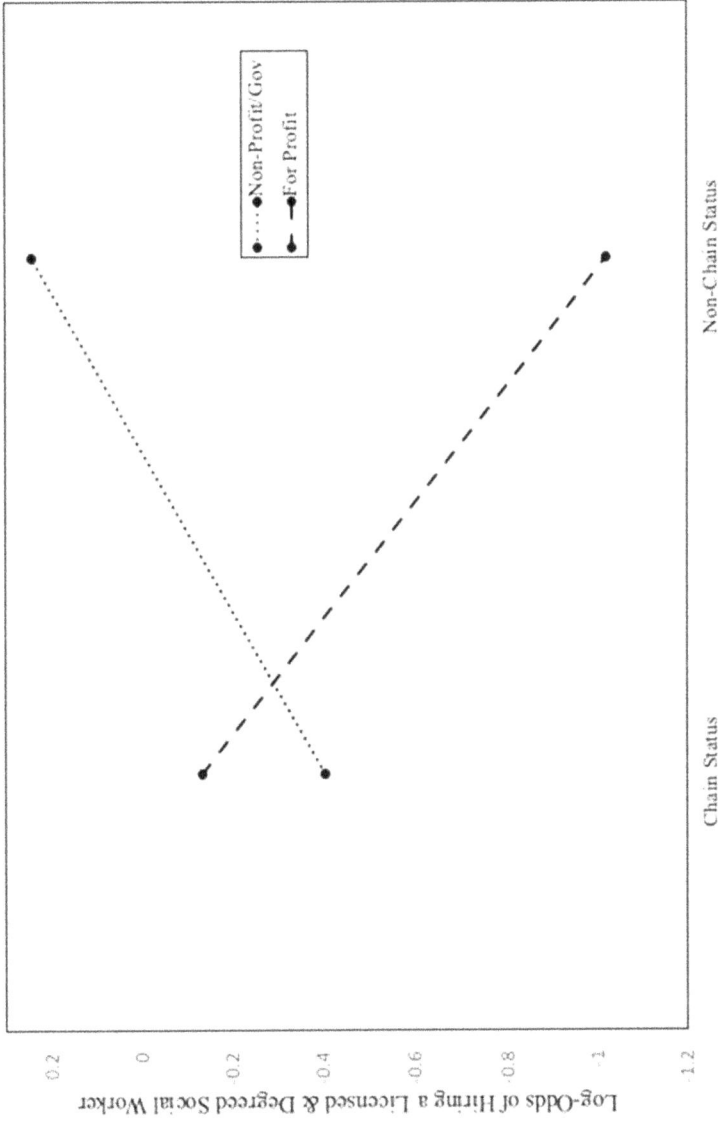

Figure 1. Interaction of chain status and ownership status among nursing homes with 120+ beds. Interaction plot of the log-odds of hiring a licensed and degreed social worker at nursing homes with 121 or more beds. The interaction indicates that, at higher levels of bed size (i.e., 121 or more beds), non-chain and nonprofit or government owned nursing homes are more likely to hire a degreed and licensed social worker.

interaction of chain status, ownership type, and nursing home bed size begin to separate, the three-way interaction is provided graphically in Figure 1. The interaction indicates that at the highest levels of bed size (i.e., 121 or more beds) non-chain and nonprofit or government-owned nursing homes were more likely to hire a degreed and licensed social worker as social services director. Conditional effects of ownership type and chain status positively, significantly interacted with the nursing homes containing 120+ beds ($\chi^2(1)$ = 6.22; log odds = 1.53; $p < .05$). The conditional interaction further supports the interpretation that the nursing homes with more than 120 beds moderates the likelihood of hiring a licensed and degreed social worker given the condition of the nursing home being not-for-profit or government-owned and not being a part of a chain. This result translates into an increased likelihood of 362% (OR = 4.62) among not-for-profit, non-chain nursing homes with 120 + beds employing a licensed and degreed social worker compared to nursing homes with 120+ beds that are part of a for-profit chain. Among nursing homes with fewer than 120 beds, those with less than 60 beds were least likely to employ a licensed and degreed social worker, regardless of region, county, or RUCC.

Discussion

This is the first study since 2006 to report data collected from a nationally representative sample of nursing home social services directors about their departments. Our first aim was to characterize the social services workforce and the second, to compare the 2019 and the 2006 workforces. As was the case in 2006, most nursing homes do employ at least one social services staff person, at least part time. Social services departments are small; in about half of the homes in the sample, there was only one person in the social services department. There is still too little gender and ethnic diversity among this workforce with most directors reported being women and white. There was an increase in social services directors with a master's degree in social work (17% in 2006 and 28% in 2019). Almost half (47%) of 2019 social services directors (including staff members without a social work degree) report having a state-issued license or certificate in social work compared to 39% in 2006. A quarter of the respondents reported their age as 55 or older which implies a large turn-over in the nation's nursing home social services workforce over the next decade. This turn-over may be hastened by the COVID-19 pandemic. One third of the sample reported 15 or more years' experience in nursing home social services. While salaries for directors have increased since 2006, 80% of social services directors who work full-time reported earning less than 60,000 USD per year. The median salary was between 40,000 and 49,000 USD. This is lower than the median salary of 67,370 USD for registered nurses working in nursing home in 2018 (Bureau of Labor Statistics, 2018) and closer to the 2018 median salary for nursing home licensed practical nurse (LPN's) of 48,330. USD

Our third and final aim was to identify the characteristics of nursing homes that are most likely to employ a social services director with both a social work education and license. In other words, we sought to identify nursing homes that employ social services directors who meet the NASW professional standards. About one-third (37%) of nursing homes in this study employ a person with both a social work degree (BSW or MSW) and a social work license/certification as social services director. Our analyses determined that larger nursing homes were more likely to hire degreed and licensed social workers. Among nursing homes with more than 120 beds, not-for-profit, nursing homes that were not part of a chain were far more likely to employ a degreed and licensed social worker as social services director compared with the same sized for-profit chain counterparts. The NASW standards for social work practice in nursing homes include a preference for social services directors to have earned an MSW. Less than one-third of the 2019 sample met the criteria of having an MSW, two-thirds of whom were licensed, therefore one-in-five (20.8%) of the nation's nursing home social services directors meet the *preferred* NASW standards to serve as the director of social services in the nursing home setting. (Social services directors with a bachelor's degree in social work also meet professional standards if they comply with state licensing requirements, and if they receive consultation from a person with an MSW.)

A limitation of the current study is the 30% response rate and the fact that data were collected only from the director of social services and not from other social services staff members. Also, nursing homes in the Midwest are slightly over-represented in the sample.

Over 40% of nursing homes have a nonsocial worker as social services director, in direct opposition to national professional standards and possibly in violation of many states' practice and title protection laws. It can be argued that this is also in opposition to federal law because although CMS has invented its own unique definition of a "qualified social worker" to be used in the case of nursing homes serving older adults and persons with disabilities, CMS also requires certified nursing homes to hire professional staff in keeping with professional standards and state law. CMS's own definition is at odds with professional standards and some state laws when it comes to determining who is qualified to be a social worker in a nursing home. CMS rules are also at odds with evidence from social services directors themselves (including respondents in this study and in the 2006 study) who reported being able to meet the psychosocial needs of far fewer than 120 residents (Bern-Klug et al., 2021).

In most nursing homes in the US, the social worker is the only staff person with the expertise to anticipate psychosocial needs of residents–including residents with dementia, assess psychosocial needs, develop a care plan that takes into account psychosocial needs, and evaluate whether the care plan interventions are making a difference. Furthermore, recent CMS rules now require nursing homes to provide culturally competent care that is trauma informed. A social work education, including continuing education requirements that accompany licensure, prepare social workers in both culturally competent care and trauma informed care.

The Code of Federal Regulations clearly states that Medicare/Medicaid nursing homes must employ staff that meet professional standards. The Code of Federal Regulations then present a completely unique definition of a professional social worker, a definition that is at odds with professional standards, and not used in other Medicare/Medicaid settings. In other words, despite the fact that the professional practice of social work is licensed in every state, and title or practice protection is in every state, and the NASW decades ago developed professional standards for social work practice in nursing homes, CMS has invented its own definition of social work, applied only in the nursing home setting, which includes people who have not earned a social work degree as "qualified social workers." It is not appropriate for the government to dilute professional standards in a setting that primarily cares for older adults.

Unlike all other Medicare/Medicaid certified settings, federal regulations in the nursing home context use the terms "social services" and "social work" interchangeably, which is confusing because social work, unlike social services, is a profession with a code of ethics, state licensure, and a rigorous educational preparation (including practicum) at the bachelors and masters level in schools accredited by the Council on Social Work Education. Allowing nonsocial workers to practice as social workers makes it difficult for residents, families, fellow staff members, and medical directors to know what they can count on in terms of psychosocial care.

For the benefit of nursing home residents, their families, and fellow staff members, we strongly recommend CMS put aside its idiosyncratic and minimalist operationalization of a "qualified social worker" and uphold professional standards by requiring a social work degree and license in order to practice as a social worker in a nursing home. In the nine states that do not license social workers at the bachelor's level, an MSW should serve as a consultant to the baccalaureate social worker

Meeting residents' psychosocial care needs is an important aspect of quality of life. It is not possible for one social worker to address the psychosocial needs of 120+ residents and maintain strong relationships with their family members. We recommend the development of a realistic staffing ratio. We recommend additional research on psychosocial needs of residents, and effective psychosocial interventions. Our final recommendation is a call for research in which the unit of analysis is the interdisciplinary team. The literature is silent on the impact on residents when the entire interdisciplinary staff is well qualified and responsible for a reasonable number of residents. While disciple-specific research continues to be needed, research on strong interdisciplinary teams in nursing homes is also called for because the needs of residents exceed the skills and expertise of any one discipline.

Acknowledgment

Special thanks to Lisa Halm-Werner, Iowa Social Science Research Center and Haley Arkfeld, School of Social Work.

Disclosure statement

Review process blinded from Editor-in-Chief on this manuscript

Funding

This study was made possible through the generous funding of the RRF Foundation for Aging.

ORCID

Mercedes Bern-Klug (iD) http://orcid.org/0000-0001-6546-6141
Nancy Kusmaul (iD) http://orcid.org/0000-0003-2278-8495

References

Association of Social Work Boards. (2018). *U.S. social work regulations and licensure exemptions*. Association of Social Work Boards. Retrieved June 16, 2020, from https://www.aswb.org/wp-content/uploads/2018/02/Social-work-licensing-exemptions-1.24.18-finalformat.pdf

Bern-Klug, M., Byram, E., Steinberg, N. S., Garcia, H. G., & Burke, K. (2018). Nursing home residents' legal access to onsite professional psychosocial care: Federal and state regulations do not meet minimum professional social work standards. *The Gerontologist, 58*(4), e260–e272. Retrieved June 14, 2020, from. https://doi.org/10.1093/geront/gny053

Bern-Klug, M., Byram, E., Steinberg, N.S., Garcia, H.G., & Burke, K. (2018). Nursing home residents' legal access to onsite professional psychosocial care: Federal and state regulations do not meet minimum professional social work standards. *The Gerontologist,58*(4), e260–e272. doi:10.1093/geront/gny053.

Bern-Klug, M., Carter, K., & Wang, Y. (2021). *More evidence that federal regulations perpetuate unrealistic nursing home social services staffing ratios.* (Under review). Journal of Gerontological Social Work.

Bern-Klug, M., Kramer, K. W. O., Chan, G., Kane, R., Dorfman, L., & Saunders, J. (2009). Characteristics of nursing home social services directors: How common is a degree in social work? *JAMDA, 10*(1), 36–44. https://doi.org/10.1016/j.jamda.2008.06.011

Bern-Klug, M., Kramer, K. W. O., Sharr, P., & Cruz, I. (2010). Nursing home social services directors' opinions about the number of residents they can serve. *Journal of Aging & Social Policy, 22*(1), 33–52. https://doi.org/10.1080/08959420903396426

Bonifas, R. P. (2016). *Bullying among older adults: How to recognize and address an unseen epidemic.* Health Professions Press.

Bureau of Labor Statistics. (2018). *National occupational employment and wages.* Bureau of labor statistics. Retrieved February 28, 2020, from https://www.bls.gov/ooh/healthcare/licensed-practical-and-licensed-vocational-nurses.htm#tab-4. BLS RNs in NF/SNF https://www.bls.gov/oes/current/oes291141.htm. BLS LPN in nursing care facilities: https://www.bls.gov/oes/current/oes292061.htm

CMS. (2017). *State operations manual, Appendix PP - guidance to surveyors for long term care facilities.* Center for Medicare and Medicaid Services. Retrieved August 10, 2020, from: https://www.cms.gov/Regulations-and-Guidance/Guidance/Manuals/downloads/som107ap_pp_guidelines_ltcf.pdf

Code of Federal Regulations. 2020. *Title 42: Public HealthPART 483—REQUIREMENTS FOR STATES AND LONG TERM CARE FACILITIESSubpart B—Requirements for Long Term Care Facilities.* U.S. Government. Retrieved June 19, 2020, from https://www.ecfr.gov/cgi-bin/retrieveECFR?gp=&SID=a00abdc8033ee43c2b5f2df2890054b2&mc=true&n=pt42.5.483&r=PART&ty=HTML

Craney, T. A., & Surles, J. G. (2002). Model-dependent variance inflation factor cutoff values. *Quality Engineering, 14*(3), 391–403. https://doi.org/10.1081/QEN-120001878

Drageset, J., Dysvik, E., Espehaug, B., Natvig, G. K., & Furnes, B. (2015). Suffering and mental health among older people living in nursing homes - A mixed-methods study. *Peer Journal, 3*, e1120. https://doi.org/10.7717/peerj.1120

Federal Register. (2016). *Medicare and medicaid programs; reform of requirements for long-term care facilities.* RIN 0938-AR61, p. 68801hosmer. U.S. Government. Retrieved August 18, 2020, from https://www.govinfo.gov/content/pkg/FR-2016-10-04/pdf/2016-23503.pdf

Florida Statutes. (2020). *Title XXXIII, regulation of professions and occupations, chapter 491, clinical, counseling, and psychotherapy services, 491.016, Social Work, title use.* State of Florida. Retrieved October 1, 2020, from http://www.leg.state.fl.us/statutes/index.cfm?App_mode=Display_Statute&URL=0400-0499/0491/0491.html

Harris-Kojetin, L., Sengupta, M., Lendon, J. P., Rome, V., Valverde, R., & Caffrey, C. (2019). Long-term care providers and services users in the United States, 2015–2016. National Center for Health Statistics. *Vital Health Statistics, 3*(43), 22. Retrieved July 14, 2020, from https://www.cdc.gov/nchs/data/series/sr_03/sr03_43-508.pdf

Hayes, A. F. (2017). *Introduction to mediation, moderation, and conditional process analysis: A regression-based approach.* Guilford publications.

Hosmer, D. W., Lemeshow, S., & Sturdivant, R. X. (2013). *Applied logistic regression* (3rd ed.). Wiley.

NASW. (2003) *NASW standards for social work services in long-term care facilities.* National Association of Social Workers. Retrieved June 14, 2020, from https://www.socialworkers.org/LinkClick.aspx?fileticket=cwW7lzBfYxg%3D&portalid=0

Roberts, A. R., Smith, A. C., & Bowblis, J. R. (2019). *Impact of social service staffing on nursing home quality and resident outcomes.* Scripps Gerontology Center Report. https://miamioh.edu/cas/academics/centers/scripps/research/publications/2019/03/social-service-staffing-nh-quality.html

Simons, K., Connolly, R. P., Bonifas, R. P., Allen, P., Bailey, K., Downes, D., & Galambos, C. (2012). Psychosocial assessment of nursing home residents via MDS 3.0: Recommendations for social service training, staffing, and roles in interdisciplinary care. *JAMDA, 13*(2), 190.e9-190.e15. https://doi.org/10.1016/j.jamda.2011.07.005

Zhang, N. J., Gammonley, D., Paek, S. C., & Frahm, K. (2008). Facility service environments, staffing, and psychosocial care in nursing homes. *Health Care Financing Review, 30*(2), 5–17. https://www.ncbi.nlm.nih.gov/pmc/articles/PMC4195051/pdf/hcfr-30-02-005.pdf

Serious Mental Illness in Nursing Homes: Roles and Perceived Competence of Social Services Directors

Denise Gammonley, Xiaochuan Wang, Kelsey Simons, Kevin M. Smith, and Mercedes Bern-Klug (iD)

ABSTRACT
Providing nursing home psychosocial care to persons with serious mental illnesses (SMI) requires understanding of comorbidities and attention to resident rights, needs and preferences. This quantitative study reports how 924 social service directors (SSDs) taking part in the National Nursing Home Social Service Director survey identified their roles and competence, stratified by the percentage of residents with SMI. More than 70% of SSDs, across all categories of homes, reported the social services department was "always" involved in conducting depression screening, biopsychosocial assessments and PASRR planning. SSDs in homes with lower concentrations of residents with SMI reported less involvement in anxiety screening. Those employed in homes with higher concentrations of residents with SMI reported lower involvement conducting staff interventions for resident aggression or making referrals. More than one-fifth of SSDs lacked confidence in their ability to compare/contrast dementia, depression, and delirium or to develop care plans for residents with SMI. SSDs' perceived competence in developing care plans for residents with SMI was associated with education and involvement in care planning. About one-quarter of social services directors reported not being prepared to train a colleague on how to develop care plans for residents with SMI. Training in SMI could enhance psychosocial care.

Data obtained from the Minimum Data Set (MDS) 3.0 in 2018 indicate that 20% of the US nursing home population has serious mental illness (SMI) (e.g., bipolar disorder, schizophrenia, or a psychotic disorder) (PASRR Technical Assistance Center, 2020). Providing quality care to residents with serious mental illnesses (SMI) presents nursing homes with challenges in providing individualized care, specialized services, and appropriate staff training (Kaldy, 2018; Muralidharan et al., 2019). Assessments are required upon admission to ensure the nursing home meets both medical and mental illness needs of prospective residents (PASRR Technical Assistance Center, 2016). Care planning must account for medical and behavioral health comorbidities. For incoming residents with SMI specialized services may be required to address mood and behavioral concerns. Vigilant attention to protecting resident rights including the right to community integration must also be provided (Olmstead v. L.C., 1999).

Social service providers are essential to delivering psychosocial care to residents with SMI. They provide screening and assessing for behavioral health issues, conducting biopsychosocial assessments, serving as resident and family advocates. Facilitating staff training, care planning and consulting with mental health providers for residents with SMI may require further tasks or training focused on behavioral health. The purpose of this study is to describe characteristics of nursing homes serving residents with SMI and social services department involvement in delivering psychosocial care to residents with these disorders. The study will examine the perceived roles and competence of social service directors who participated in the 2019 National Nursing Home Social Services Director Survey. This nationally representative sample of social service directors from U.S. certified nursing homes responded to questions about their involvement in tasks and responsibilities, barriers to delivering care, perceived competence to train social service staff, departmental staffing, and job satisfaction.

Background

The minimum federal standards for approving state Medicaid plans require individual screening of all prospective nursing home residents for mental illness. A Preadmission Screening Resident Review (PASRR) Level I screen is used to determine if a prospective resident has a mental illness. If positive, a Level II screen verifies the presence of a defined mental disorder and determines appropriateness for nursing home or community care based on the duration of the most recent illness, and the level of recent functional impairment. The regulatory environment for PASRR varies as states can establish broader definitions of SMI, operate their PASRR programs differently–including setting timelines for re-review of residents, and pay for required specialized services for residents with SMI from any source other than the standard nursing facility rate. Accordingly, state regulatory guidelines for residents with SMI differ with a majority of states having little to no attention to mental illness in their nursing home regulations (Street et al., 2013).

Serious mental illness and quality of care in nursing homes

Having SMI or being cared for in a nursing home where many residents have these conditions is associated with poorer care quality. Residents with SMI are more likely to be concentrated in for-profit facilities having a higher Medicaid census (Jester et al., 2020) and in facilities with overall poorer quality (Jester et al., 2020; Rahman et al., 2013). They are also admitted to homes with more deficiencies (Li et al., 2011) and to lower quality homes for post-acute nursing home stays (Temkin-Greener et al., 2018). Within Veterans Affairs nursing homes, facilities having higher concentrations of residents with SMI are more likely to use physical restraints (Kim et al., 2013). Despite the high need for psychosocial care, facilities having a higher proportion of residents with SMI also employ fewer social services staff in comparison to facilities with a smaller concentration of residents with SMI (Jester et al., 2020).

Psychosocial needs of nursing home residents with SMI

Complex combinations of medical, social, rehabilitation and behavioral health interventions characterize the essential services and supports necessary for residents with SMI. The burden of living with SMI encompasses medical comorbidity, functional impairments often preventing independent living, self-management of medical conditions and limits on the availability of social support or sustained family involvement over the adult life course (K. A. Aschbrenner et al., 2011a; Bartels et al., 2018). Persons with SMI experience premature mortality influenced by medical conditions, socioeconomic and health disparity factors (Druss et al., 2011). Due to these risk factors, people with SMI who are admitted to nursing homes are often younger than persons with other conditions who are admitted (Andrews et al., 2009). Despite the Olmstead mandate to return persons with disabilities to the community (Olmstead v. L.C., 1999), there is a greater likelihood of a long-term stay among residents with SMI (K. Aschbrenner et al., 2011b). This may reflect the lack of options in the community.

Biopsychosocial assessment, referral, and interventions for resident behavioral health concerns are essential components of delivering quality psychosocial care upon admission and throughout a stay in the nursing home. Referrals for specialized behavioral health services may be required upon admission due to PASRR Level II requirements or later as part of care planning in response to changing resident needs. Suicidal ideation, both at admission and discharge for post-acute residents, and for residents with long-term stays, is more prevalent among residents with a SMI diagnosis as documented in the MDS (Temkin-Greener et al., 2020). A recent study also found aggressive behaviors occur among only 9.3% of residents with SMI diagnoses in the absence of dementia. However, 23.1% of residents with co-morbid SMI diagnoses and dementia exhibited aggressive behavior in the nursing home (Cen et al., 2018). The overlap between dementia behaviors and behaviors associated with SMI diagnoses underscores the importance of having adequately prepared social service providers capable of assessing behavioral concerns, consulting with geriatric behavioral health professionals to facilitate and monitor referrals, and training staff members to address behavior concerns.

Responsiveness to depression, suicidal ideation and aggression is especially important for residents with SMI (Rahman et al., 2013). Nursing home care quality and staffing is linked to the presence of behavioral health concerns. For example, the odds of a nursing home having more severe depression, aggression, and suicidal ideation among its residents has recently been associated with inadequate community service coordination, limited staff education, and high staff turnover (Orth et al., 2020).

To adequately address disparities affecting residents with SMI psychosocial care should also address vulnerabilities related to social support and end-of-life care. Psychosocial care should include helping residents with SMI maintain, or sometimes reestablish, family relationships and provide support and counseling to manage relationships within the nursing home. Residents with SMI are less likely to have an advanced care plan (Cai et al., 2011) or receive palliative care (Donald & Stajduhar, 2019) and will benefit from social service providers providing counseling, decision-making support and advocacy at the end of life.

Social service roles in caring for residents with SMI

Behavioral health services based on an assessment and care plan provided by a sufficient number of adequately trained staff are required to ensure residents attain or maintain the highest practicable physical, mental and psychosocial well-being (Requirements for Centers for Medicare and Medicaid Services, 2016). Medically related social services are required to be part of this care through participation in interdisciplinary care planning, conducting biopsychosocial and behavioral health assessments, providing person-centered counseling and support, and delivering advocacy on behalf of residents (Centers for Medicare and Medicaid Services, 2017).

Social service staffing is a cost-efficient strategy to improve the quality of care and quality of life for residents in nursing homes (Bowblis & Roberts, 2020). Among post-acute care residents, improvements in resident behavioral symptoms and use of antipsychotic medications have been noted when more-qualified social service staff are available (Roberts et al., 2020). While the broad range of core functions provided by social services in nursing homes has been described (Bern-Klug & Kramer, 2013), the roles and responsibilities among providers in homes where residents with SMI are concentrated is not as well understood. Anecdotally, social services has been described as the discipline helpful for addressing challenging resident behaviors and networking in the community to provide appropriate resources for residents with SMI (Kaldy, 2018). However, the degree of preparation of social service directors to undertake the careful assessments of behavioral symptoms, comorbidities, and contextual factors needed to achieve that goal is not well understood.

Further, it is not clear if social services directors feel prepared to respond directly, and/or by training fellow staff members, to respond to the unique psychosocial care needs for residents with SMI.

As residents with SMI are at especially high risk for poor outcomes due to health disparities it is important to understand the extent to which the perceived competence of social service directors aligns with their roles and responsibilities in caring for residents with SMI. The first aim of the study is to describe the roles and competence of social service directors in providing care across facilities considering the percentage of residents with SMI. The second aim is to understand the associations between facility and SSD characteristics, social services departmental roles and self-perceived social services directors' competence in SMI care planning.

Method

Data and sample

This study is a secondary data analysis of the 2019 National Nursing Home Social Services Director survey (NNHSSD), a nationally representative survey of nursing home social services directors in the United States. A random sample of 3,650 was drawn from the 15, 577 Medicare and/or Medicaid certified nursing homes nationwide, identified using the Nursing Home Compare publicly available dataset. Out of the initial random sample, 3,067 nursing homes were found to have at least one social services employee at the time of study as identified through phone verification process. Of those, 924 participated in the survey online or on paper, yielding a response rate of 30%.

The 2019 NNHSSD survey contained 185 questions, including SSD's demographic and professional characteristics, structures and roles of social services department, perceived barriers to care, perceived competence, employment benefits, job satisfaction, and resident characteristics. Facility characteristics, such as ownership status, chain affiliation, facility size, were obtained through Centers for Medicare & Medicaid Services (CMS) Provider of Services (POS) Current Files and matched to each respondent using unique participant IDs. The study was performed in compliance with the University of Iowa institutional review board.

Measures

Social services roles in planning and providing care
SSDs were asked to use a 4-point scale (1 = social services is never involved to 4 = social services is always involved) to rate the extent to which the social services department was involved in 1) biopsychosocial assessment; 2) screen for anxiety; 3) screen for depression; 4) create/develop individual care plans addressing psychosocial needs; 5) provide counseling (psychotherapy)

sessions; 6) refer residents to a mental health professional; 7) participate in developing level 2 PASRR care plans; and 8) plan staff intervention to prevent/minimize aggressive behaviors. Responses coded as "This is not done at our facility" were treated as missing values. Responses were constructed into three categories (never/rarely involved, usually involved, or always involved)."

Perceived competence

Perceived competence was assessed by asking respondents the preparation time they need to "provide one-on-one training to a social services colleague about . . . ." in 1) conducting biopsychosocial assessment; 2) developing care plans for residents with SMI; 3) comparing/contrasting dementia, depression, and delirium and anticipate common psychosocial needs; 4) assessing psychosocial needs of residents under age 60, develop care plan, connect with community resources; 5) requesting a "mental health consultation" with mental health professionals; and 6) describing who may benefit from counseling services, how to arrange services, and how services will be paid for. Responses ranged from 1 = "could do without prep time" to 4 = "not able to do". Two response options ("could do without prep time" and "would need up to 2 hours of prep time") were combined and coded as 1 (able to do with minimal preparation). The remaining two answer options were combined into 0 (unable to do or would need up to 10 hours of preparation).

Percentage of residents with serious mental illness (SMI)

SSDs were asked to estimate "what percentage of your nursing home residents have a serious mental illness such as schizophrenia, bi–polar disorder, serious depression or serious PTSD". Response options ranged from 1 = less than 10% of residents with SMI to 4 = 50% or more of residents with SMI. In this study, responses were constructed into 3 categories where low = less than 10%, medium = 10–49%, high = 50% or more.

Social services directors' demographic and professional characteristics

Demographic characteristics assessed included gender, age, and race. SSDs' professional characteristics included years of experience in nursing home social services (<1 year, 1–3 years, 4–9 years, 10–15 years, and 15 years or more), educational attainment (< 4 year degree, Bachelor's degree, and Master's degree), having a social work degree (yes/no), and having a social work license/certification (yes/no).

Facility characteristics

Facility characteristics included ownership status (for profit, government, and nonprofit), program participation (Medicare only, Medicaid only, and Medicare and Medicaid), metropolitan location (yes/no), chain affiliation (yes/no), number of certified beds (less than 60, 60-120, 121 or more), whether the facility contracted with an outside mental health provider (yes/no), and whether mental health services were provided off-site to residents (yes/no).

Data analyses

Demographic and professional characteristics of SSDs and facility information were analyzed using descriptive statistics. Chi-square tests were performed to evaluate social services roles and perceived competence differences, respectively, among nursing homes with different categories of percentage of residents with SMI. To address aim 2, we first used Chi–square tests and Fisher's Exact tests to examine whether association existed between social services roles and SSDs' perceived competence in developing care plans for residents with SMI, in the full sample and stratified by percentage of residents with SMI, respectively. We further performed a logistic regression to examine the association between SSD characteristics, facility characteristics, social services roles, and perceived competence in SMI care plan development. Odds ratios (ORs) and 95% confidence intervals (95% CIs) were reported. Statistical analyses were conducted using SPSS, Version 26.

Results

Sample description

Table 1 presents the demographic and professional backgrounds of SSDs, as well as facility characteristics. Most SSDs surveyed were female (92.1%), and White/Caucasian (86.8%). Approximately half of the respondents were 35-54 years old (47.8%), reported bachelor's degree as highest education level (49.0%), had social work degrees (57.9%), and possessed a Social Work license/certification (47.4%). Most nursing homes were for–profit (62.7%), participated in both Medicare and Medicaid programs (95.2%), were in metropolitan areas (66.9%), were chain affiliated (58.1%), and had 60-120 certified beds (52.9%).

SSD reported a broad distribution of residents with SMI; 368 SSDs (40.4%) estimated that less than 10% of their residents had a SMI, 424 SSDs (46.5%) reported their facility having 10%-49% residents with SMI, whereas the remaining 13.1% reported greater than 50% of their residents had SMI. Most nursing homes (88.8%) contracted with external providers for mental health and/or behavioral health services directly provided to residents (including but not limited to residents with SMI). Less than one-fifth of the mental health services were provided off-site (17.9%).

Social services roles by resident SMI percentage

Table 2 presents the extent to which SSDs reported departmental role involvement in the eight activities pertinent to planning and providing mental health

Table 1. Descriptive statistics of study variables (n = 924).

Variables	N	%
SSD Demographics and professional characteristics		
Gender		
Male	69	7.5
Female	845	92.1
Diverse/Other	3	0.3
Age		
18–34	257	28.1
35–54	437	47.8
55 and up	220	24.1
Race		
White/Caucasian	802	86.8
Other	122	13.2
Years of experience in NHSS		
Less than 1 year	68	7.4
1–3 years	175	19.0
4–9 years	244	26.5
10–15 years	147	16.0
15 years or more	287	31.2
Educational attainment		
<4 year degree	142	15.6
Bachelor's degree	447	49.0
Master's degree	323	35.4
Social Work degree (Yes BSW and/or MSW)	528	57.9
Social Work license/certification (Yes)	429	47.4
Facility and resident characteristics		
Ownership status		
For profit	572	62.7
Government	77	8.4
Nonprofit	264	28.9
Program Participation		
Medicare only	20	2.2
Medicaid only	24	2.6
Medicare and Medicaid	869	95.2
In metropolitan area (Yes)	611	66.9
Chain status (Yes)	530	58.1
Number of total beds		
Less than 60	182	19.9
60-120	483	52.9
121 or more	248	27.2
Contracts with MH provider (Yes)	810	88.8
MH services provided off-site to residents (Yes)	163	17.9
Percentage of residents with SMI		
Less than 10%	368	40.4
10%–49%	424	46.5
50% or more	119	13.1

NH = nursing home; SS = social services; MH = mental health; SMI = serious mental illness.

care. Of those reporting that such activities were conducted in the facilities, more than half of SSDs reported social services was "always involved" in seven activities, including developing individual care plans for psychosocial needs (88.0%). Social service directors reported biopsychosocial assessments (87.6%), screening for depression (76.6%), referring residents to a mental health professional (76.3%), developing level 2 PASARR care plans (72.4%), developing staff interventions to prevent/minimize aggressive behaviors (63.2%), and screening for anxiety (58.8%), regardless of the percentage of residents with SMI.

Table 2. Roles in planning & providing care by percentage of residents with serious mental illness (SMI).

Social Services Roles in Planning & Providing Care	Overall	Percentage of Residents with SMI			$\chi^2(df)$	p
		Low (<10%)	Medium (11–49%)	High (50%+)		
Biopsychosocial assessment					2.45(4)	.65
Rarely/never involved, n (%)	38 (4.4)	13 (3.7)	21 (5.2)	4 (3.5)		
Usually involved, n (%)	70 (8.1)	31 (8.9)	28 (6.9)	11 (9.6)		
Always involved, n (%)	761 (87.6)	305 (87.4)	356(87.9)	100 (87.0)		
Individual care plans for psychosocial needs					10.48(4)	<.05
Rarely/never involved, n (%)	34 (3.8)	14 (3.8)	12 (2.9)	8 (6.8)		
Usually involved, n (%)	74 (8.2)	35 (9.6)	25 (6.0)	14 (12.0)		
Always involved, n (%)	795 (88.0)	317 (86.6)	383 (91.2)	95 (81.2)		
Screen for anxiety					9.91(4)	<.05
Rarely/never involved, n (%)	200 (22.7)	90 (25.4)	82 (19.9)	28 (24.4)		
Usually involved, n (%)	163 (18.5)	77 (21.8)	68 (16.5)	18 (15.7)		
Always involved, n (%)	518 (58.8)	187 (52.8)	262 (63.6)	69 (60.0)		
Screen for depression					8.93(4)	.06
Rarely/never involved, n (%)	99 (11.0)	33 (9.0)	48 (11.4)	18 (15.4)		
Usually involved, n (%)	112 (12.4)	57 (15.6)	45 (10.7)	10 (8.6)		
Always involved, n (%)	692 (76.6)	276 (75.4)	327 (77.9)	89 (76.1)		
Refer to MH professional					20.43(4)	<.001
Rarely/never involved, n (%)	55 (6.1)	23 (6.3)	17 (4.0)	15 (12.8)		
Usually involved, n (%)	159 (17.6)	76 (20.9)	73 (17.3)	10 (8.6)		
Always involved, n (%)	688 (76.3)	264 (72.7)	332 (78.7)	92 (78.6)		
Develop level 2 PASRR care plans					1.43(4)	.84
Rarely/never involved, n (%)	144 (17.0)	51 (15.5)	71 (17.5)	22 (19.3)		
Usually involved, n (%)	90 (10.6)	38 (11.6)	40 (9.9)	12 (10.5)		
Always involved, n (%)	614 (72.4)	240 (73.0)	294 (72.6)	80 (70.2)		
Provide counseling (psychotherapy) sessions					3.52(4)	.47
Rarely/never involved, n (%)	324 (41.0)	132 (42.4)	152 (41.0)	40 (36.7)		
Usually involved, n (%)	161 (20.4)	69 (22.2)	68 (18.3)	24 (22.0)		
Always involved, n (%)	306 (38.7)	110 (35.4)	151 (40.7)	45 (41.3)		
Staff intervention to prevent/minimize aggressive behaviors					13.34(4)	<.01
Rarely/never involved, n (%)	101 (11.2)	42 (11.5)	37 (8.8)	22 (18.6)		
Usually involved, n (%)	232 (25.6)	106 (29.0)	100 (23.7)	26 (22.0)		
Always involved, n (%)	572 (63.2)	217 (59.5)	285 (67.5)	70 (59.3)		

Table 2 also presents distribution of social services role involvement by percentage of residents with SMI. Chi-square tests identified four activities in which social services involvement varied across nursing homes with different percentages of residents with SMI, including developing individual care plans (χ^2 = 10.48, 4, p < .05), screening for anxiety($\chi2$ = 9.91,4, p < .05), referring to a mental health professional (χ^2 = 20.43, 4, p < .001) and developing staff intervention to prevent aggressive behaviors(χ^2 = 13.34, 4, p < .01) . The extent to which social services was involved in creating/developing individual care plans to address resident psychosocial needs differed significantly among facilities according to the concentration of residents with SMI (p< .05). Post hoc comparisons using Bonferroni corrected alpha levels suggested that high involvement of social services (i.e. always involved) was more prevalent among nursing homes with medium concentration of residents with SMI (91.2%), as compared to those with low (86.6%) or high (81.2%) percentages of residents with SMI.

A smaller percentage (52.8%) of SSDs from nursing homes with low concentration of residents with SMI reported that social services was always involved in screening for anxiety, compared to those with medium (63.6%) and high (60.0%) concentrations of SMI residents (p< .05). Additionally, social services involvement in referring residents to mental health professionals (p< .001) and developing staff interventions to prevent or minimize aggressive behaviors (p< .01) also varied significantly by percentage of residents with SMI. Occasional or no involvement of social services in mental health referrals and staff intervention for aggressive behaviors were more frequently reported in facilities with a high percentage of residents with SMI (12.8% and 18.6%, respectively), as compared to those had low and medium percentages of residents with SMI. Moreover, 8.6% of SSDs from nursing homes having high concentration of residents with SMI reported that social services was usually involved in the referral of residents to mental health professionals, a significantly lower percentage than that reported in nursing homes with low (20.9%) and medium (17.3%) concentrations of SMI residents (Table 2).

Perceived competence by resident SMI percentage

As presented in Table 3, irrespective of percentage of residents with SMI, at least 70% of SSDs perceived themselves as being able to train others without preparation or with no more than 2 hours of preparation time on all the six topics examined, ranging from requesting mental health consultation (92.9%) to developing care plans for residents with SMI (74.0%). Results from Chi-square tests indicated that SSDs' perceived competence in developing care plans for residents with SMI concerns varied across different categories of percentage of residents with SMI (p< .01). SSDs in

Table 3. Perceived competence by percentage of residents with serious mental illness (SMI).

Perceived Competence	Percentage of Residents with SMI				χ2(df)	p
	(n) Overall	Low	Medium	High		
Conduct biopsychosocial assessment					0.61(2)	.74
Able to do with minimal prep, n (%)	710 (80.3)	279 (79.0)	337 (81.2)	94 (81.0)		
Unable to do or require extensive prep, n (%)	174 (19.7)	74 (21.0)	78 (18.8)	22 (19.0)		
Develop care plans for residents with SMI					10.73(2)	<.01
Able to do with minimal prep, n (%)	654 (74.0)	242 (68.2)	324 (78.5)	88 (75.9)		
Unable to do or require extensive prep, n (%)	230 (26.0)	113 (31.8)	89 (21.6)	28 (24.1)		
Compare/contrast dementia, depression, and delirium and anticipate common psychosocial needs					0.08(2)	.96
Able to do with minimal prep, n (%)	678 (76.6)	272 (76.6)	316 (76.3)	90 (77.6)		
Unable to do or require extensive prep, n (%)	207 (23.4)	83 (23.4)	98 (23.7)	26 (22.4)		
Assess psychosocial needs of residents under age 60, develop care plan, connect with community resources					2.21(2)	.33
Able to do with minimal prep, n (%)	715 (80.6)	279 (78.6)	344 (82.7)	92 (79.3)		
Unable to do or require extensive prep, n (%)	172 (19.4)	76 (21.4)	72 (17.3)	24 (20.7)		
Request a MH consultation with mental health professionals					0.70(2)	.71
Able to do with minimal prep, n (%)	825 (92.9)	331 (92.7)	389 (93.5)	105 (91.3)		
Unable to do or require extensive prep, n (%)	63 (7.1)	26 (7.3)	27 (6.5)	10 (8.7)		
Describe who may benefit from counseling services, how to arrange services, how services will be paid for					2.81(2)	.25
Able to do with minimal prep, n (%)	807 (90.9)	328 (91.1)	381 (91.8)	98 (86.7)		
Unable to do or require extensive prep, n (%)	81 (9.1)	32 (8.9)	34 (8.2)	15 (13.3)		

MH = mental health; SMI = Serious mental illness. Low = < 10%, Medium = 10-49%, High = 50% or more.

nursing homes with low percentage of residents with SMI (31.8%) tend to perceive themselves as being unable to or requiring extensive preparation (up to ten hours) to train others to develop care plans for residents with SMI. Whereas SSDs of facilities with medium proportion of residents with SMI tend to report being able to provide training with no or minimal preparation time (78.5%).

Association between social service roles and perceived competence for developing care plans

As shown in Table 4, regardless of the percentage of residents with SMI in a facility, social services directors' SSDs report of the departmental role in screening for anxiety (*p* < .01), creating/developing individual care plans for resident psychosocial needs (*p* < .001), and providing mental health referrals (*p* < .01), were significantly associated with their perceived competence in developing care plans for residents with SMI. As reported in more detail below, results are organized by the percentage of residents with SMI.

Among nursing homes with low percentage (less than 10%) of residents with SMI, social services involvement in individual care plan development for psychosocial needs was found associated with SSD's perceived competence in developing care plans for residents with SMI (*p* < .01). In nursing homes with a low percentage of residents with SMI where social services was always involved in the creation or development of individual care plan for

Table 4. Social services directors' report of departmental roles and self–competence in SMI care plan development by percentage of residents with SMI.

| | Percentage of Residents with SMI | | | | | | | |
| | Overall, n (%) | | Low, n (%) | | Medium, n (%) | | High, n (%) | |
Perceived competence	Able with minimal prep	Unable/need extensive prep	Able with minimal prep	Unable/need extensive prep	Able with minimal prep	Unable/need extensive prep	Able with minimal prep	Unable/need extensive prep
Screen for anxiety								
Rarely/never involved	125 (64.4)	69 (35.6)	52 (59.1)	36 (40.9)	56 (71.8)	22 (28.2)	17 (60.7)	11 (39.3)
Usually involved	114 (73.5)	41 (26.5)	47 (66.2)	24 (33.8)	53 (79.1)	14 (20.9)	14 (82.4)	3 (17.6)
Always involved	391 (77.3)	115 (22.7)**	133 (72.7)	50 (27.3)	204 (79.7)	52 (20.3)	54 (80.6)	13 (19.4)
Individual care plans for psychosocial needs								
Rarely/never involved	14 (43.8)	18 (56.3)	4 (33.3)	8 (66.7)	6 (50.0)	6 (50.0)	4 (50.0)	4 (50.0)
Usually involved	44 (63.8)	25 (36.2)	18 (52.9)	16 (47.1)	17 (77.3)	5 (22.7)	9 (69.2)	4 (30.8)
Always involved	593 (76.3)	184 (23.7)***	220 (71.4)	88 (28.6)**	300 (79.8)	76 (20.2)	73 (78.5)	20 (21.5)
Refer to MH professional								
Rarely/never involved	31 (58.5)	22 (41.5)	13 (56.5)	10 (43.5)	11 (68.8)	5 (31.3)	7 (50.0)	7 (50.0)
Usually involved	104 (68.0)	49 (32.0)	49 (68.1)	23 (31.9)	49 (69.0)	22 (31.0)	6 (60.0)	4 (40.0)
Always involved	514 (76.6)	157 (23.4)**	177 (69.1)	79 (30.9)	264 (81.2)	61 (18.8)*	73 (81.1)	17 (18.9)*
Staff intervention to prevent/minimize aggressive behaviors								
Rarely/never involved	64 (65.3)	34 (34.7)	23 (56.1)	18 (43.9)	26 (74.3)	9 (25.7)	15 (68.2)	7 (31.8)
Usually involved	158 (72.1)	61 (27.9)	66 (67.3)	32 (32.7)	73 (76.0)	23 (24.0)	19 (76.0)	6 (24.0)
Always involved	428 (76.3)	133 (23.7)	151 (70.9)	62 (29.1)	224 (80.0)	56 (20.0)	53 (77.9)	15 (22.1)

Note. MH = mental health; SMI = serious mental illness. *p< .05; **p< .01; ***p< .001 Low = < 10%, Medium = 10-49%, High = 50% or more.

psychosocial needs, 71.4% of SSDs reported being able to train others to develop care plans for residents with SMI with no or minimal preparation.

In nursing homes with medium concentrations of residents with SMI, the degree of social services involvement in mental health referral was associated with perceived competence in care plan development for residents with SMI ($p< .05$). SSDs from these medium SMI facilities who reported social services was always involved in referring residents to mental health professionals perceived themselves as being more competent (i.e. able to do without prep or with up to 2 hours prep time, 81.2%) rather than requiring extensive prep time or couldn't do at all (18.8%).

Among nursing homes with high concentrations of residents with SMI, the extent to which social services was involved in mental health referral was significantly associated with perceived competence in care plan development for residents with SMI ($p< .05$). SSDs who reported social services was always involved in mental health referral tended to perceive themselves being able to train others on this topic with no or minimal preparation (81.1%), rather than needing more than 10 hours of preparation time or not able to do at all (18.9%; Table 4).

Table 5 presents the results of a logistic regression model conducted to examine the association between facility and SSD characteristics, social service role involvement, and SSDs' perceived competence in developing SMI care plans. As shown in Table 5, SSDs who reported social services was rarely or never involved in individual care plans for psychosocial needs were less likely to perceive being able to train others on SMI care plan development with minimal preparation (OR = 0.23, 95% CI [0.09, 0.60], $p< .01$), as compared to those who report social services being always involved in this role. SSDs from facilities with medium concentration (10%-49%) of SMI residents were more likely to perceive competence in SMI care planning (OR = 1.50, 95% CI [1.04, 2.16], $p< .05$), comparing those from low SMI concentration facilities. Additionally, SSDs with less than 1 year of experience in nursing home social services were less likely (OR = 0.46, 95% CI [0.23, 0.91], $p< .05$) to self–report competence in SMI care plan development, as compared to those with 4-9 years of experience. Educational attainment also emerged as a significant factor. SSDs whose highest education level was less than bachelor's degree (OR = 0.47, 95% CI [0.25, 0.89], $p< .05$), and those whose highest degree was bachelor's (OR = 0.64, 95% CI [0.43, 0.97], $p< .05$), were less likely to perceive themselves as being able to train others on SMI care planning with no or minimal preparation, comparing with their counterparts with Master's degree.

Discussion

To address disparities in quality of care and quality of life among residents with SMI social service departments must be adequately resourced and trained to

Table 5. Results of logistic regression on self–competence in SMI care plan development.

Variables		OR (95% CI)
Gender (Female)	Male	0.80 (0.43, 1.52)
	Diverse/Other	0.46 (0.03, 7.39)
Age (18-34)	35-54	0.66 (0.40, 1.09)
	55 and up	0.66 (0.41, 1.08)
Race (White/Caucasian)	Other	0.91 (0.53, 1.57)
Years of experience in NHSS (4-9 years)	Less than 1 year	0.46 (0.23, 0.91) *
	1-3 years	0.83 (0.51, 1.37)
	10-15 years	1.40 (0.80, 2.45)
	15 years or more	1.37 (0.84, 2.24)
Educational attainment (Master's degree)	<4 year degree	0.47 (0.25, 0.89) *
	Bachelor's degree	0.64 (0.43, 0.97) *
Social Work degree (Yes)	No	1.26 (0.81, 1.95)
Social Work license/certification (Yes)	No	1.06 (0.73, 1.54)
Ownership type (For profit)	Government	0.85 (0.45, 1.61)
	Non-profit	0.79 (0.52, 1.18)
Program participation (Medicare and Medicaid)	Medicare only	2.62 (0.55, 12.42)
	Medicaid only	0.44 (0.16, 1.18)
In metropolitan area (Yes)	No	0.88 (0.60, 1.30)
Chain status (Yes)	No	0.72 (0.50, 1.04)
Bed size (121 or more)	<60 beds	1.00 (0.56, 1.78)
	60-120	0.89 (0.58, 1.38)
Contracts with MH provider (Yes)	No	0.73 (0.44, 1.22)
MH services provided off-site to residents (No)	Yes	1.26 (0.80, 1.98)
Percentage of residents with SMI (<10%)	10%-49%	1.50 (1.04, 2.16) *
	50% or more	1.38 (0.79, 2.42)
Screen for anxiety (Always involved)	Rarely/never involved	0.80 (0.51, 1.23)
	Usually involved	1.10 (0.69, 1.75)
Individual care plans for psychosocial needs (Always involved)	Rarely/never involved	0.23 (0.09, 0.60) **
	Usually involved	0.64 (0.34, 1.19)
Refer to MH professional (Always involved)	Rarely/never involved	0.89 (0.42, 1.89)
	Usually involved	0.79 (0.50, 1.26)
Staff intervention to prevent/minimize aggressive behaviors (Always involved)	Rarely/never involved	1.28 (0.67, 2.46)
	Usually involved	0.90 (0.60, 1.36)

NH = nursing home; SS = social services; MH = mental health; SMI = serious mental illness; OR = Odds Ratio; CI = confidence interval; $*p < .05$; $**p < .01$; $***p < .001$.

deliver psychosocial care competently. Assessment and care planning are two essential roles for social services in nursing homes that are mandated by law. Competent attention to the unique needs of residents with SMI requires specialized knowledge about psychiatric disorders, comorbidities, rights and resident preferences. Not surprisingly, SSDs in this survey reported the provision of biopsychosocial assessment and individual care planning to address psychosocial needs as endorsed roles where they were always or usually involved. It did not vary across the percentage of residents with SMI in the nursing home.

However, notable role differences were identified among the SSDs working in nursing homes with a high proportion of residents with SMI. Those working in a nursing home with a high percentage of residents with SMI were more likely to indicate that their department was only sometimes or never involved in referring a resident to a mental health professional or conducting a staff intervention to prevent or minimize aggressive behaviors. This lack of involvement may reflect overall poor quality in nursing homes serving high concentrations of residents with SMI. There is a greater likelihood of residents with SMI being admitted to poorer performing nursing homes (Li et al., 2011) and to have worse care outcomes (McGarry et al., 2019). Inadequate social services staffing may further contribute to this lack of involvement. Staffing may affect the overall availability of social services or reduce opportunities to engage in those roles. In a recent analysis social services staffing levels were noted to be lower in nursing homes with higher concentrations of residents with SMI compared to nursing homes with a small concentration of residents with SMI (Jester et al., 2020). Alternatively, nursing homes where more residents have SMI may be better prepared to offer regular consultations from mental health professionals reducing the need for SSDs to make outside referrals. Nursing homes where there are more residents with SMI may also be more likely to have nursing assistants who are more comfortable in delivering interventions for aggressive behaviors (Molinari et al., 2008).

Our findings indicate two additional areas where social service directors need support to improve their confidence to train others in delivering psychosocial care for residents with SMI. Two roles where more than one-fifth of SSDs, regardless of the concentration of residents with SMI, were not confident in their competence are in distinguishing dementia, depression and delirium (23.4% unable to do or requiring extensive preparation) and in developing care plans for residents with SMI (26.0% unable to do or requiring extensive preparation). Lack of confidence in care planning for residents with SMI was most apparent among SSDs employed in facilities with a low percentage of residents with SMI. Almost one-third (31.8%) reported being unable to train on care planning for SMI residents. Lack of confidence is especially concerning given the recently identified 77% growth in prevalence over ten years of nursing home residents with SMI (Hua et al., 2020). This trend suggests social service departments are more often being called upon to assess, develop individualized care plans, and facilitate referrals for increasing numbers of residents with SMI in all nursing homes, regardless of the proportion of residents with SMI.

We identified a contribution of educational attainment to SSD self-competence in care planning which complements recent work by Roberts et al. (2020). Their study linked the presence of qualified social workers (defined as having staff meeting the CMS educational requirement for a bachelor's degree) with improved facility performance in addressing behavioral symptoms and use of antipsychotics. In our study both SSDs who reported attaining the bachelor's degree, and those with less than a four-year degree, were less confident in their care planning competence for residents with SMI compared to SSDs with master's degrees.

Study limitations

This investigation is exploratory focusing on associations between SSD and facility characteristics including the percentage of residents with SMI, social services roles, and perceived competence. Our focus was limited to the SSD and did not consider the role of social work trainees or other social work staff members in care planning or implementation. It is possible that in self-reporting the percentage of nursing home residents with SMI that SSDs may have over or underestimated the number of residents they are caring for with serious mental illness. Our emphasis was on assessment, planning and mental illness intervention roles (screening, assessments, care planning, responding to aggression) but we did not include attention to other social service roles (such as assisting with substance abuse concerns, advanced care planning, discharge planning, facilitating relationships in the community and with family). These roles are also of great importance in caring for residents with SMI.

Training recommendations and implications

Clearly recognizing distinctions between dementia, depression, and screening for anxiety to anticipate and plan for resident psychosocial needs is essential for social services staff. However, differential diagnosis of symptoms, particularly when residents have a co-occurring SMI disorder, can be especially challenging (Felmet et al., 2011). To respond effectively to the complex and sometimes overlapping symptoms presenting in residents with SMI it is particularly important for social services staff to receive specialized training. The availability of qualified social workers trained in behavioral health contributes to nursing homes' satisfaction with their ability to deliver behavioral health services (Orth et al., 2019). Muralidharan et al. (2019) have noted an emphasis of training long-term care staff on dementia but a lack of focus on training regarding the needs of residents with SMI. Included in their curricular recommendations are a focus on understanding how the key features of the progression of cognitive decline differ among persons with SMI. Simulation has been used as an acceptable method to train social work students to recognize geriatric depression (Gellis & Kim, 2017). Web-based and simulation training may also be an accessible approach for training nursing home social workers about SMI as well (Molinari et al., 2017).

Competent behavioral health practice by nursing home social services requires skill in behavior management, building relationships, as well as in using redirection (Myers et al., 2019). Responding to aggression requires additional specialized skill. Bonifas (2015) highlights the importance of competent assessment focused on investigating environmental and other causal factors and the essential role of the social worker in facilitating collaborative staff relationships to manage aggression. Training may help promote confidence in social service departments to respond to aggression by delivering staff education.

The degree of involvement of social workers in care planning meetings is likely to vary as CMS regulations do not mandate the involvement of social services as a member of the interdisciplinary care planning team (Centers for Medicare and Medicaid Services, 2017). Understanding the nature of "involvement" of social services in care planning is an important area for further research. The varied psychosocial needs of residents with SMI underscores the importance of actively engaging social workers in interdisciplinary care team meetings for residents with SMI. Care planning requires careful assessment of preferences and goals related to discharge, community reintegration, family involvement and end-of-life care. Moreover, social services should serve as an advocate for SMI residents promoting the protection of their right to be discharged and reintegrated into the community.

Overall, findings from this exploration of social services departmental roles and director's self-perceived competence suggests training in mental health assessments, especially for anxiety, depression, dementia and delirium as well as in developing care plans for residents with SMI and responding to aggression would be valuable. Training for those SSDs with less than master's level education and limited experience will be especially important. Training alone will be insufficient to ensure adequate psychosocial care for residents with SMI. Policy reforms are needed to ensure adequate social services staffing, inclusion of social service providers as key contributors to care planning teams, and increased access to appropriate behavioral health services for residents.

Funding

This study was made possible through the generous funding of the RRF Foundation for Aging.

ORCID

Mercedes Bern-Klug ⓘ http://orcid.org/0000-0001-6546-6141

References / *Referencias*

Andrews, A. O., Bartels, S. J., Xie, H., & Peacock, W. J. (2009). Increased risk of nursing home admission among middle aged and older adults with schizophrenia. *American Journal of Geriatric Psychiatry*, *17*(8), 697–705. https://doi.org/10.1097/JGP.0b013e3181aad59d

Aschbrenner, K., Grabowski, D. C., Cai, S., Bartels, S. J., & Mor, V. (2011b). Nursing home admissions and long-stay conversions among persons with and without serious mental illness. *Journal of Aging and Social Policy*, *23*(3), 286–304. https://doi.org/10.1080/08959420.2011.579511

Aschbrenner, K. A., Cai, S., Grabowski, D. C., Bartels, S. J., & Mor, V. (2011a). Medical comorbidity and functional status among adults with major mental illness newly admitted to nursing homes. *Psychiatric Services*, *62*(9), 1098–1100. https://doi.org/10.1176/ps.62.9.pss6209_1098

Bartels, S. J., Dimilia, P. R., Fortuna, K. L., & Naslund, J. A. (2018). Integrated care for older adults with serious mental illness and medical comorbidity evidence-based models and future research directions. *Psychiatric Clinics North America*, *41*(1), 153–164. https://doi.org/10.1016/j.psc.2017.10.012

Bern-Klug, M., & Kramer, K. W. O. (2013). Core functions of nursing home social services departments in the United States. *Journal of the American Medical Directors Association*, *14*(1), 75.e1-75.e7. https://doi.org/10.1016/j.jamda.2012.09.004

Bonifas, R. P. (2015). Resident-to-resident aggression in nursing homes: Social worker involvement and collaborat ion with nursing colleagues. *Health & Social Work*, *40*(3), e101–e109. https://doi.org/10.1093/hsw/hlv040

Bowblis, J. R., & Roberts, A. R. (2020). Cost-effective adjustments to nursing home staffing to improve quality. *Medical Care Research and Review*, *77*(3), 274–284. https://doi.org/10.1177/1077558718778081

Cai, X., Cram, P., & Li, Y. (2011). Origination of medical advance directives among nursing home residents with and without serious mental illness. *Psychiatric Services*, *62*(1), 61–66. https://doi.org/10.1176/ps.62.1.pss6201_0061

Cen, X., Li, Y., Hasselberg, M., Caprio, T., Conwell, Y., & Temkin–Greener, H. (2018). Aggressive behaviors among nursing home residents: Association with dementia and behavioral health disorders. *Journal of the American Medical Directors Association*, *19*(12), 1104–1109.e4. https://doi.org/10.1016/j.jamda.2018.09.010

Centers for Medicare and Medicaid Services. (2016). *Requirements for states and longterm care facilities, 42 C.F.R. § 483.40 - Behavioral health services.* https://www.govinfo.gov/app/details/CFR-2019-title42-vol5/CFR-2019-title42-vol5-sec483-40/summary

Centers for Medicare and Medicaid Services. (2017). *Appendix PP. Guidance to surveyors for long-term care facilities. State operations manual.* https://www.cms.gov/Regulations-and-Guidance/Guidance/Manuals/downloads/som107ap_pp_guidelines_ltcf.pdf

Donald, E. E., & Stajduhar, K. I. (2019). A scoping review of palliative care for persons with severe persistent mental illness. *Palliative and Supportive Care*, *17*(4), 479–487. https://doi.org/10.1017/S1478951519000087

Druss, B. G., Zhao, L., Von Esenwein, S., Morrato, E. H., & Marcus, S. C. (2011). Understanding excess mortality in persons with mental illness: 17-year follow up of a nationally representative US survey. *Medical Care*, *49*(6), 599–604. https://doi.org/10.1097/MLR.0b013e31820bf86e

Felmet, K., Zisook, S., & Kasckow, J. W. (2011). Elderly patients with schizophrenia and depression: Diagnosis and treatment. *Clinical Schizophrenia & Related Psychoses*, *4*(4), 239–250. https://doi.org/10.3371/CSRP.4.4.4

Gellis, Z. D., & Kim, E. G. (2017). Training social work students to recognize later-life depression: Is standardized patient simulation effective? *Gerontology & Geriatrics Education*, *38*(4), 425–437. https://doi.org/10.1080/02701960.2017.1311882

Hua, C. L., Cornell, P. Y., Zimmerman, S., Winfree, J., & Thomas, K. S. (2020). Trends in serious mental illness in US assisted living compared to nursing homes and the community: 2007-2017. *The American Journal of Geriatric Psychiatry*. Advance online publication. https://doi.org/10.1016/j.jagp.2020.09.011

Jester, D. J., Hyer, K., & Bowblis, J. R. (2020). Quality concerns in nursing homes that serve large proportions of residents with serious mental illness. *The Gerontologist*, *60*(7), 1312–1321. https://doi.org/10.1093/geront/gnaa044

Kaldy, J. (2018). When mental illness and aging make nursing homes necessary: What next? *Caring for the Ages*, *19*(5), 1–11. https://doi.org/10.1016/j.carage.2018.04.001

Kim, H. M., Banaszak-Holl, J., Kales, H., Mach, J., Blow, F., & McCarthy, J. F. (2013). Trends and predictors of quality of care in VA nursing homes related to serious mental illness. *Medical Care*, *51*(8), 659–665. https://doi.org/10.1097/MLR.0b013e318293c28d

Li, Y., Cai, X., & Cram, P. (2011). Are patients with serious mental illness more likely to be admitted to nursing homes with more deficiencies in care? *Medical Care, 49*(4), 397–405. https://doi.org/10.1097/MLR.0b013e318202ac10

McGarry, B. E., Joyce, N. R., McGuire, T. G., Mitchell, S. L., Bartels, S. J., & Grabowski, D. C. (2019). Association between high proportions of seriously mentally ill nursing home residents and the quality of resident care. *Journal of the American Geriatrics Society, 67*(11), 2346–2352. https://doi.org/10.1111/jgs.16080

Molinari, V., Hobday, J., Roker, R., Kunik, M., Kane, R. A., Kaas, M., Mehrotra, C., Williams, C., Robbins, J. C., & Dobbs, D. (2017). Impact of serious mental illness online training for certified nursing assistants in long term care. *Gerontology & Geriatrics Education, 38*(4), 359–374. https://doi.org/10.1080/02701960.2016.1188811

Molinari, V., Merritt, S., Mills, W., Chiriboga, D., Conboy, A., Hyer, K., & Becker, M. (2008). Serious mental illness in Florida nursing homes: Need for training. *Gerontology & Geriatrics Education, 29*(1), 66–83. https://doi.org/10.1080/02701960802074321

Muralidharan, A., Mills, W. L., Evans, D. R., Fujii, D., & Molinari, V. (2019). Preparing long-term care staff to meet the needs of aging persons with serious mental illness. *Journal of the American Medical Directors Association, 20*(6), 683–688. https://doi.org/10.1016/j.jamda.2019.03.018

Myers, D. R., Rogers, R. K., LeCrone, H. H., & Kelley, K. (2019). The behavioral health role in nursing facility social work. *Journal of Applied Gerontology, 38*(8), 1063–1095. https://doi.org/10.1177/0733464817733103

Olmstead v. L.C., 527 U.S. 581. (1999). https://www.loc.gov/item/usrep527581/

Orth, J., Li, Y., Simning, A., & Temkin-Greener, H. (2019). Providing behavioral health services in nursing homes is difficult: Findings from a national survey. *Journal of the American Geriatrics Society, 67*(8), 1713–1717. https://doi.org/10.1111/jgs.16017

Orth, J., Li, Y., Simning, A., & Temkin-Greener, H. (2020). Severe behavioral health manifestations in nursing homes: Associations with service availability? *Journal of the American Geriatrics Society, 68*(11), 2643–2649. https://doi.org/10.1111/jgs.16772

PASRR Technical Assistance Center. (2016). *PASRR in plain english.* https://www.pasrrassist.org/resources/PASRR-in-Plain-English

PASRR Technical Assistance Center. (2020). *2019 PASRR national report: A review of pre-admission screening and resident review (PASRR) programs.* https://www.pasrrassist.org/resources/2019-PASRR-National-Report

Rahman, M., Grabowski, D. C., Intrator, O., Cai, S., & Mor, V. (2013). Serious mental illness and nursing home quality of care. *Health Services Research, 48*(4), 1279–1298. https://doi.org/10.1111/1475-6773.12023

Roberts, A. R., Smith, A. C., & Bowblis, J. R. (2020). Nursing home social services and post-acute care: Does more qualified staff improve behavioral symptoms and reduce antipsychotic drug use? *Journal of the American Medical Directors Association, 21*(3), 388–394. https://doi.org/10.1016/j.jamda.2019.07.024

Street, D., Molinari, V., & Cohen, D. (2013). State regulations for nursing home residents with serious mental illness. *Community Mental Health Journal, 49*(4), 389–395. https://doi.org/10.1007/s10597-012-9527-9

Temkin-Greener, H., Campbell, L., Cai, X., Hasselberg, M. J., & Li, Y. (2018). Are post-acute patients with behavioral health disorders admitted to lower-quality nursing homes? *American Journal of Geriatric Psychiatry, 26*(6), 643–654. https://doi.org/10.1016/j.jagp.2018.02.005

Temkin-Greener, H., Orth, J., Conwell, Y., & Li, Y. (2020). Suicidal ideation in US nursing homes: Association with individual and facility factors. *American Journal of Geriatric Psychiatry, 28*(3), 288–298. https://doi.org/10.1016/j.jagp.2019.12.011

Social Services Involvement in Care Transitions and Admissions in Nursing Homes

Colleen Galambos, Laura Rollin, Mercedes Bern-Klug ⓘ, Mike Oie, and Eric Engelbart

ABSTRACT

Care transitions (CT) are critical junctures in the healthcare delivery process. Effective transitions reduce the need for subsequent transfers between healthcare settings, including nursing homes. Understanding social services (SS) involvement in these processes in nursing homes is important from a quality and holistic care perspective. Using logistic regression, this study examines structural and relational factors identified with higher involvement of SS in care transitions and admissions. SS directors from 924 nursing homes were evaluated in relation to SS involvement in care transitions and admissions processes. Results suggest the level of SS involvement in care transitions and admissions are associated with structural factors such as size of facility, geographical location, ratio of FTE's to beds, ownership status, and standalone SS departments, as well as relational factors, including perceptions and utilization of SS staff by facility leadership, coworkers, and family. Additionally, SS staff with higher levels of expertise and with social work degrees are less involved in admissions tasks.

Introduction

The role of social services (SS) in care transitions and the potential to improve care captured professional and national interests. Care transitions refer to changes in a person's health delivery that necessitates changes in healthcare settings and health practitioners in response to changes in conditions and care needs (Smith et al., 2014). Literature supports the notion that the complexities of working with older adults in a variety of settings requires a systems level rethinking about care delivery (Golden, 2011). Research demonstrates the value of social work involvement in care transitions (CT) based on the complex nature of these processes and the unique skills set of social workers (Alvarez et al., 2016, Bern -Klug et al., 2021; Golden, 2011; Lipani, Holster & Bussey, 2015; Sussman & Dupuis, 2014; Weerahandi et al., 2015). Specifically, social workers provide additional support to residents, family and staff across organizational settings which allows for stronger communication across settings and smoother transitions (Sussman & Dupuis, 2014).

Social work strengthens care transitions

Social workers create improved outcomes in CT based on their holistic perspective and person-centered approach to care, a departure from traditional models. Resident and family psychosocial needs are a vital component of the holistic, person-centered approach utilized by social workers (Fields et al., 2012). In particular, the development of a social work care plan takes into consideration the interplay between psychological and social factors of the client and their caregivers, as well as the resources necessary to provide care, which contrasts the disease-centered approach of traditional medical models (Fabbre et al., 2011).

Based on their person-centered care approach, social workers are aptly equipped to take on higher-difficulty CT which require conflict resolution and problem-solving. Social work skills include mediation and counseling, a necessary asset when developing a discharge care plan that involves multiple healthcare professionals, community providers, and the patient and family. Knowledge of systems, community resources, and brokerage skills facilitates connections to needed services and support networks. For these traits and others, social work expertise is recognized as a vital component to the facilitation of successful CT (Sims-Gould et al., 2015; Sussman & Dupuis, 2014).

Communication is central to social work led transitions. Models of care emphasizing social work focus on the ability to develop relationships with patients, caregivers, and providers of health care and other supportive services while providing psychosocial support (Alvarez et al., 2016; Fabbre et al., 2011). Research examining the contributions of social workers with other discharge planners indicates that social workers were identified with the tasks of mental health assessment, family counseling, education, and community outreach (Holliman et al., 2003). Broadly, social workers provide a variety of services during transitional care including assessment, discharge planning, staff collaboration, individual and family counseling, and education (Altfeld et al., 2013; Auerbach et al., 2007). The impact of social services involvement in care transitions includes reductions in 30-day readmission rates (Barber et al., 2015; Weerahandi et al., 2015), 60-day hospitalization rates (Weerahandi et al., 2015), and 90-day hospitalization rates (Weerahandi et al., 2015). These reductions in hospitalization rates resulted in inpatient cost savings (Weerahandi et al., 2015). Other studies highlight the importance of a social work led transitional care model, PACT, in reducing inpatient utilization and emergency department visits, while increasing follow-up discharge appointments (Lipani et al., 2015), and the Bridge Model in improving the quality of transitional care for older adults and reducing hospital readmissions (Alverz et al., 2016).

The admissions process in nursing home facilities is one component of CT and is often emphasized in skilled nursing facilities (SNFs). Nursing home admissions begin with a preadmission process where decisions are made to pursue nursing home care. Activities at this point include pre- admission assessments, communication, and coordination of the pending admission. On the day of admission, activities include initial assessments, admissions paperwork, and helping the resident and family to adjust to their new environment. These activities require a professional to support the resident who possesses strong communication and advocacy skills. Due to patient commitment and advocacy, strong communication skills, and understanding of complex psychosocial factors, social workers are often tasked with intake and assessment during admissions (Fields et al., 2012; Simons et al., 2012). Social workers are also tasked with pre-admission education and addressing the psychosocial needs of residents and family during the admissions process (Fields et al., 2012; Simons et al., 2012). One study of the admission process in assisted living facilities emphasizes the important role of social workers in preadmission education and in addressing psychosocial needs (Fields et al., 2012) to a smooth transition process. As residents enter an unfamiliar living environment, social workers teach and encourage self-advocacy, an important skill as residents learn how to navigate their new environment and advocate for their social and care needs (Bronstein et al., 2015).

Reasons for poor transitions

The most prevalent types of transitions faced by older adults are admissions to long-term care (LTC) facilities, discharges from acute care hospitalizations, and discharges from skilled nursing facilities. These situations pose significant risks for adverse outcomes due to changes in healthcare status and care plans and adjusting to new environments (Gruneir et al., 2012). Discharges from SNF's back into the community pose challenges as residents work to achieve independence with limited resources available to support the change (Popejoy, et al., 2020).

Readmissions may occur as the result of unsatisfactory transitional care. Specifically, barriers to care and lack of follow-up after discharge are linked to higher readmission rates and contribute to 30-day readmission rates among Medicare beneficiaries of nearly 20% (Jencks et al., 2009). Poor CT leading to rehospitalizations may be attributed to inadequate management and sharing of information. In response, some care coordination models use social work principles emphasizing gathering, organizing, and managing critical information to avoid future readmissions or negative health outcomes (Alvarez et al., 2015; Golden, 2011; Lipani et al., 2015; Sims-Gould et al., 2015; Weerhandi et al., 2015). Also, research links nurse staffing ratios in long-term care facilities to quality of care and transition processes (Fitzpatrick & Tzouvara, 2019). One study revealed an association between high social services case-loads and lower psychosocial care provision (R. Bonifas, 2008).

Social work services in nursing homes

In 1981, the National Association of Social Workers (NASW) published standards for social work practice in nursing homes. This was a first step to defining the social work role in LTC facilities (NASW, 1981). With these standards, attention was directed toward developing criteria for acceptable practice in LTC facilities. These standards were followed up with another NASW led initiative in 1988 to identify and develop clinical indicators for measuring social work performance in nursing homes (Vourlekis et al., 1992).

In 2003, these standards were updated and included a description of key areas of practice for social workers:

"Social work services in long-term care settings focus on several key areas, including the social and emotional impact of physical or mental illness or disability, the preservation and enhancement of physical and social function-ing, the promotion of the conditions essential to ensure maximum benefits from long-term health-care services, the prevention of physical and mental illness and increased disability, and the promotion and maintenance of phy-sical and mental health and an optimal quality of life (NASW, 2003, p. 11)." In refining these standards, practice parameters within an interdisciplinary set-ting were established.

The work on professional standard setting has continued with efforts to quantify psychosocial care in nursing home settings. Simons et al. (2012) outlines 15 best practices roles for social workers in the delivery of psychoso-cial care, including assessment, education, care planning, crisis intervention, advocacy and participation in care transitions. The identification of best practice roles is a first step in quantifying psychosocial care activities and their impact on resident care.

In addition to defining how psychosocial care is implemented in nursing homes, quality psychosocial care is link to the use of qualified staff. In the delivery of psychosocial care in nursing homes, there is evidence that the quality of psychosocial care is stronger in facilities that utilized highly qualified social service staff (Zhang et al., 2008).

Additionally, Roberts et al. (2020) analysis of the presence of social service staff on resident outcomes indicates that stronger resident outcomes are associated with reducing behavioral symptoms and avoiding the use of psychotropic medications. R. P. Bonifas (2015) outlines the important role of social workers in addressing resident to resident aggression in nursing homes including assessment, intervention, and collaborative strategies, emphasizing social worker – nurse collaborations. Most recently, Berne Klug and Beaulieu (2020) outline the critical contributions social workers make in nursing home settings including connecting residents with families, reviewing advance directive documentation with residents, and providing psychosocial counseling and support to residents impacted by loss and isolation.

Functions of social services departments

The Nursing Home Reform Act of 1987, set the current standard for social work staffing (Code of Federal Regulations, 1987). This Act recognized the importance of social services and mandated that the social service needs of residents be met in Medicare and Medicaid certified nursing homes. It required facilities with more than 120 beds to employ a full time qualified social worker. For nursing homes with beds under that amount, the social service needs of residents can be met through other staffing qualifications and arrangements.

Bern -Klug et al., (2013) identified a core set of functions in which SS departments are usually or always involved. Top functions reported by SS directors included activities related to the CT process such as involvement in discharge planning, transfers, orientation of resident and family to the facility, and family counseling. Less reported functions are coordination of admissions paperwork and screening processes.

A review of the literature indicates that social workers and SS departments in nursing homes provide an important role in CT. This study was propelled by the current health environment which drives increasing care transition demands on nursing homes, and an-emphasis on medical care in facilities, while de-emphasizing psychosocial care (Zúñiga et al., 2015). To find out more about what factors may be linked to high involvement of social workers in CT, the authors analyzed factors that supported involvement in admissions and CT for social workers, and social service staff. Data was obtained from a national sample of SNF's, whose respondents were directors of social service department. The study methods and analysis will be explained in the next sections.

Methods

Data

The included analysis uses quantitative cross-sectional survey data from a nationally representative sample of 924 nursing home social services directors. This analysis is part of a larger study examining the roles and responsibilities of social services in nursing homes throughout the United States.

Nursing homes were excluded from the study if they did not employ at least one SS staff member.

In January 2019, a random sample of 3,650 Medicare and/or Medicaid certified nursing homes listed on the December 2018 Center for Medicare and Medicaid Services (CMS) Nursing Home Compare Database (available to the public on the CMS website) was drawn from an existing pool of 15, 557 nursing homes. Out of this pool, it was determined through phone calls to each of the 3,650 facilities that 3,067 employed a SS director at the time of the study. During the screening phone call, the SS director's e-mail and name were requested by personnel from this study. Invitations to participate in the study were then e-mailed to the SS director. If no e-mail address was available, or no e-mail response received, a hard copy of the invitation and survey instrument was mailed to the nursing home to the attention of the SS director. Each SS director was sent an invitation to participate in the study along with a questionnaire. Of the 3,067 nursing home SS directors invited, 924 responded to the invitation and completed the survey (536 completed the survey online and 388 completed on paper), for a response rate of 30%. Nursing home characteristics were similar between the online and paper respondents. This paper reports on the characteristics of SS staff and their facilities in relation to their role in CT including the admissions process.

Description of dependent variables

The dependent variables used in this study were comprised of a composite score of a series of questions related to the extent that social services is involved in various aspects of admissions processes or CT. Possible answers ranged from *Social services is never involved* (coded as 1) to *Social services is always involved* (coded as 4). Responses of *This is not done at our facility* were coded as missing. These variables were then categorized as binary dependent variables and given a value of *higher involvement* if the total composite score was greater than the mean score for that variable or *lower involvement* if the total composite score was less than or equal to the mean score for that variable.

The composite outcome variables were created by categorizing involvement across different categories and aggregating responses into one score for each outcome variable. We explored treating the outcomes as continuous, and decided that, while some power is lost in categorizing them, we gain a lot of practical significance in interpretation by categorizing level of involvement. Additionally, the distribution of the "involvement in care transitions" variable was highly skewed to the left, and rather than running a linear regression with an adjustment for the nonparametric distribution, we decided it was more prudent to categorize the outcome so that, relative to one another, we were able to conceptualize high and low involvement. Furthermore, the differences

Table 1. Questions Comprising the Composite Score for Level of Social Services Involvement in Admissions Processes and Care Transitions.

To what extent is social services involved?
Admissions Processes
(1) Review preadmissions documentation to determine suitability for admission
(2) Visit potential residents in the hospital or at home to assess for possible admission
(3) Explain to residents/family when and how to apply for Title 19 (Medicaid)
(4) Explain to residents/families nursing home coverage paid by Medicare, Medicare Advantage, Medigap, Medicare Savings Programs, Part D drug plan, and the VA. Also explain what is NOT covered.
(5) Coordinate the admissions paperwork
(6) As part of the admissions process, discuss tentative plans for discharge with resident/family
Care Transitions
(1) Meet with nursing and others to discuss/decide discharge plans for short-stay patients/residents (receiving post-acute/sub-acute/rehab or/skilled care)
(2) Meet with nursing and others to discuss/decide discharge plans for long-stay (long-term care) residents
(3) Meet (in-person/phone) with resident/family to discuss discharge plans, 4–7 days prior to discharge
(4) Meet (in-person/phone) with resident/family to discuss discharge plans on the discharge day
(5) Conduct at least one follow-up phone call/visit to resident's home within 7 days after discharge
(6) Help to decide when to transfer a resident to a psychiatric facility/unit for evaluation
(7) Identify long-stay (long-term care) residents who might be candidates to be discharged to the community, with services
(8) Arrange services in the community for residents who are being transferred from your facility to live in the community

between each value of the aggregate scores are not uniformly calculable, thus lending themselves to more practical interpretation as categorical variables.

Level of social services involvement in admissions processes

The level of SS involvement in admissions processes was determined by totaling the responses to six questions (Table 1). Total possible scores ranged from six to 24 for the extent to which social services is involved in admissions processes. The mean score for level of involvement in admissions processes was 16.95 (SD = 4.58). Observations with a mean composite score greater than 16.95 were considered to have social services higher involvement in admissions processes and those with a score of 16.95 or lower were considered to have lower involvement.

Level of social services involvement in care transitions

The level of SS involvement in CT was determined by totaling the responses to eight questions (Table 1). Total possible scores ranged from eight to 32 for the extent to which social services is involved in CT. The mean score for level of involvement in admissions processes was 28.97 (SD = 3.30). Observations with a mean composite score greater than 29 were considered to have higher SS involvement in CT and those with a score of 29 or lower were considered to have lower involvement.

Statistical analyses

All analyses were conducted using Stata/IC 15.1. The analyses were restricted to observations with no missing values, yielding an analytical sample size of 665. First, descriptive statistics were estimated for all variables (Table 2). Next, we fit

Table 2. Sample Characteristics of Nursing Homes and Nursing Home Social Services Directors (n = 665).

Characteristics	Percentage[a] or Mean (*SD*)
Facility characteristics	
Ownership type	
For profit	63.01
Nonprofit	28.57
Government	8.42
Number of beds	
<60	17.89
60–120	53.98
≥121	28.12
Metro area	
Metro	67.07
Non-metro	32.93
Part of chain of 2+ nursing homes	
Yes	58.80
No	41.20
Social services is its own department	
Yes	91.73
No	8.27
Number of FTE[b] positions per 100 residents	1.63 (4.58)
Percent of social services staff time spent on short-term patients	
0–24%	16.39
25–49%	27.67
50–74%	35.79
75–100%	20.15
Social services directors	
Education	
Less than 4-year college degree	16.39
Bachelor's degree	49.02
Master's degree	34.59
Has a social work degree (BSW or MSW)	
Yes	57.89
No	42.11
Holds a state license in social work	
Yes	46.77
No	53.23

Abbreviations: SD, standard deviation; FTE, full-time equivalent; BSW/MSW, Bachelor/Master of Social Work
[a]Percentages may not sum to 100 due to rounding.
[b]Includes total FTEs for up to 3 employees. If employee works ≥35 hours, FTE = 1. If employee works <35 hours, FTE = 0.5. Calculation: (total # of FTEs for all social services employees/# of beds)*100.

unadjusted and adjusted logistic regression models (Table 3) in order to estimate the strength of the associations between our independent variables of interest and each of the dependent variables. Adjusted models control for a variable that was created to measure the proportion of the total number of social services hours worked among social services employees in the facility to the number of beds at each nursing home, represented as number of FTE positions per 100 beds (henceforth referred to as FTE per 100 beds). An FTE of 1.0 was assigned to social services employees that worked greater than or equal to 35 hours per week and an FTE of 0.5 was assigned to those that worked less than 35 hours per week, for up to three social services employees in each facility. This ratio provides a cleaner measure of SS staff support that is comparable across nursing homes.

Table 3. Odds Ratios (Logistic Regression Estimates) for High Social Services Involvement in Admissions Processes and Care Transitions at Nursing Homes (n = 665).

Characteristics	Admissions Processes[a]		Care Transitions[a]	
	OR (95% CI)	P-value	OR (95% CI)	P-value
Ownership type				
For profit (ref)	1.00	-	1.00	-
Nonprofit	1.84 (1.27, 2.65)	0.001*	0.71 (0.50, 1.01)	0.060
Government	1.54 (0.85, 2.79)	0.152	0.62 (0.35,1.10)	0.101
Number of beds				
< 60	7.56 (4.09, 13.97)	<0.001*	0.76 (0.46, 1.26)	0.290
60–120	2.03 (1.38, 2.98)	<0.001*	1.00[b] (0.70, 1.43)	0.986
≥ 121 (ref)	1.00	-	1.00	-
Metro area				
Metro (ref)	1.00	-	1.00	-
Non-metro	2.13 (1.51, 3.00)	<0.001*	1.17 (0.85, 1.63)	0.339
Part of chain of 2+ nursing homes				
Yes	0.63 (0.46, 0.87)	0.005*	0.93 (0.68, 1.27)	0.653
No (ref)	1.00	-	1.00	-
SS is its own department				
Yes	0.93 (0.52, 1.66)	0.809	1.90 (1.08, 3.35)	0.027*
No (ref)	1.00	-	1.00	-
Number of FTE[c] positions per 100 beds[d]	2.00 (1.59, 2.54)	<0.001*	1.00[b] (0.86, 1.16)	0.974
75–100%	0.52 (0.31, 0.89)	0.017*	0.60 (0.36, 1.01)	0.054
Education of SS director				
Less than 4-year college degree (ref)	1.00	-	1.00	-
Bachelor's degree	0.70 (0.45, 1.10)	0.125	1.04 (0.68, 1.61)	0.845
Master's degree	0.46 (0.29, 0.74)	0.002*	1.09 (0.69, 1.72)	0.717
SS director has a social work degree (BSW or MSW)				
Yes (ref)	1.00	-	1.00	-
No	1.49 (1.08, 2.05)	0.015*	1.24 (0.91, 1.69)	0.174
Identified "social services is not represented on key committees" as a moderate to major barrier to care[e]				
Yes	0.74 (0.46, 1.19)	0.214	0.59 (0.37, 0.93)	0.024*
No (ref)	1.00	-	1.00	-
Identified "Not enough social service staff for the number of residents" as a moderate to major barrier to care				
Yes	0.98 (0.71, 1.35)	0.899	0.73 (0.53, 1.00[b])	0.047*
No (ref)	1.00	-	1.00	-
Identified "Social and emotional needs are perceived as much less important than medical and nursing needs in this facility" as a moderate to major barrier to care				
Yes	0.92 (0.67, 1.26)	0.596	0.68 (0.50, 0.93)	0.017*
No (ref)	1.00	-	1.00	-
Administrator regularly engages the expertise of SS department				
Agree	0.77 (0.43, 1.36)	0.361	2.22 (1.26, 3.92)	0.006*
Disagree (ref)	1.00	-	1.00	-
Neutral	0.75 (0.37, 1.52)	0.422	1.07 (0.53, 2.18)	0.843
Family members regularly engage the expertise of SS department				
Agree	2.76 (0.78, 9.76)	0.116	3.85 (1.05, 14.13)	0.042*
Disagree (ref)	1.00	-	1.00	-
Neutral	3.31 (0.77, 14.22)	0.108	2.71 (0.61, 11.94)	0.189
Coworkers seem to value the role of SS in resident/family care				
Agree (ref)	1.00	-	1.00	-
Disagree	0.83 (0.43, 1.61)	0.583	0.41 (0.21, 0.82)	0.011*
Neutral	1.11 (0.64, 1.93)	0.717	1.09 (0.64, 1.88)	0.747

Abbreviations: OR, odds ratio; CI, confidence interval; ref, reference group; SS, social services; FTE, full-time equivalent; BSW/MSW, Bachelor/Master of Social Work
[a]Adjusted for FTE positions per 100 residents; [b]Rounded up to 1.00
[c]Includes total FTEs for up to 3 employees. If employee works ≥35 hours, FTE = 1. If employee works <35 hours, FTE = 0.5. Calculation: (total # of FTEs for all social services employees/# of beds×100).
[d]Unadjusted; [e]n = 664; *Statistically significant at the $p < 0.05$ level.

Results

Descriptive findings

As shown in Table 2, nearly two-thirds of nursing homes included in these analyses were for-profit (63.01%) and located in a metro area (67.07%). The majority were part of a chain of two or more nursing homes (58.80%) and housed between 60 and 120 beds (53.98%). SS was its own department in 91.73% of nursing homes. SS staff at just over half (55.94%) of nursing homes spent 50% or more of their time on short-term patients. Among social services directors, 49.02% held a Bachelor's degree, 57.89% held a social work degree (Bachelor's or Master's), and 46.77% held a state license in social work. The mean number of FTE per 100 beds was 1.63 (standard deviation [SD] = 1.00).

Logistic regression results

Social services involvement in admissions processes

Table 3 reports the logistic regression results on the selected variables that show significance. We found that each one-unit increase in FTE per 100 beds was associated with a 100% increase in the odds of higher admissions processes involvement. SS involvement was more likely with these staffing patterns. After adjusting for FTE, nonprofit ownership of the nursing home was associated with 84% higher odds of higher SS involvement in admissions compared with for-profit ownership. Nonprofit ownership was associated with the likelihood of having higher social service involvement compared with for profit ownership. An association between admissions involvement and the number of beds in the facility was also revealed. Nursing homes with less than 60 beds and between 60 and 120 beds were shown to have 7.56 and 2.03 times the odds, respectively, of higher SS involvement in admissions compared with nursing homes with greater than 120 beds. Nursing homes with 120 beds or fewer had a higher likelihood of increased social service involvement in admissions compared with nursing homes with more than 120 beds. Results also revealed that the odds of higher SS involvement in admissions for nursing homes located in a non-metro was 113% higher compared with a metro area, while the odds of higher SS involvement in admissions for facilities that were part of a chain of two or more nursing homes was 37% lower compared with independent facilities. Nursing homes located in non-metro areas and independent were more likely to have higher SS involvement.

Qualifications of the SS director influences social service involvement. Nursing homes with a SS director who did not have a social work degree were associated with 49% higher odds of having higher SS involvement in admissions, while nursing homes where the director had a master's degree (in any field) were associated with 54% lower odds of having higher SS involvement in admissions. Having a social work or master's degree decreased the likelihood of increased involvement in admissions.

Nursing homes with higher SS involvement in CT were associated with 78% higher odds of also having higher SS involvement in admissions processes compared with facilities with low SS involvement in CT. Similarly, nursing homes with higher SS involvement in admissions processes were associated with 72% higher odds of also having higher SS involvement in CT compared with facilities with lower SS involvement in admissions, indicating a relationship between involvement in admissions and CT.

Social services involvement in care transitions

We found that the odds of higher SS involvement in CT for nursing homes with standalone SS departments was 90% higher compared with those without a standalone SS department.

Several relationship factors were associated with admissions and CT involvement. Nursing homes where SS directors reported that the administrator or resident family members regularly engage the expertise of the SS department were associated with 122% and 285% higher odds of having higher SS involvement in CT compared with those that did not report so. Self-reported regular engagement increased the likelihood of CT involvement.

Additionally, facilities with SS directors that did not think that their coworkers value the role of social services in resident and family care were associated with 59% lower odds of higher SS involvement in CT compared with those that did feel so. High SS involvement is less likely when it is perceived that coworkers devalue social services work.

Facilities with SS directors that identified the following as moderate to major barriers to care: "social services is not represented on key committees," "not enough social service staff for the number of residents," and "social and emotional needs are perceived as much less important than medical and nursing needs in this facility" were associated with 41%, 27%, and 32% lower odds of higher SS involvement in CT compared with facilities where these were not identified as moderate to major barriers. In other words, these barriers were associated with a lesser likelihood that social services are involved in CT.

Discussion

The results of this study indicate that there are both structural and relational factors contributing to a higher involvement of social services/social work in admissions and CT functions. For the purposes of this discussion, we define structural factors, based in organizational theory, as the economic, social, policy, and organizational environments that "structure" the context in which social services is carried out within nursing home environments.

Relational factors are based in relational theory and are defined as the inter-actions between individuals and others which incorporate how each work together. The results will be discussed using this framework. One finding related to the qualifications of the SS staff will be discussed separately.

Structural factors

The impact of structural factors has its roots in organizational theory. Classic organization theory focuses on the arrangements within a corporation includ-ing chain of command, patterns of formal authority, division of labor, and policies and procedures; in other words, how the work of the organization is arranged, and the structure developed for getting the work done. Modern revisions to organization theory recognized the influence of past goals and performance, as well as the performance of comparable organizations on organizational operations. The impact of external and environmental factors are considered structural entities that impact organizational performance. Fiscal resources and other organizational factors are managed based on per-formance opportunities such as expectations to make a profit (Haveman & Wetts, 2019).

Such structural factors as nonprofit status, government ownership, inde-pendent status, and FTE positions per 100 beds were related to higher social service involvement in nursing home admissions. This result can be explained through the philosophy of nonprofit/government organizational practices that encourage fiscal resource returning to the facility to support patient/resident care rather than used to make a profit. This practice emphasizes the value of resident care, and explains the likelihood that facilities employ and use social services to enhance resident care during admissions. This finding is supported by Harrington et al.'s (2001) research on investor ownership and quality of care which concluded that investor-owned nursing homes provide worse care than non-profit or government-owned facilities. O'Neill et al. (2003) also reported lower quality of care as measured by deficiencies in profit or pro-prietary facilities.

The higher the FTE per beds can be attributed to the fact that having a robust employee base increases the capacity to adequately support psycho-social factors that emerge during the admissions process. Certainly, higher staffing is linked to higher quality of care (O'Neill et al., 2003). Harrington et al. (2000) research revealed that nursing homes with lower staffing, including social workers, had higher deficiencies. Finally, Bonifas (2008) finding that higher social service caseloads reduced psychosocial care sup-port is a reminder of the importance of staffing in delivering psychosocial care.

Another structural factor that emerged as a significant relationship with higher social service involvement in admissions was the size of the facility.

Smaller facilities, or nursing homes with 120 beds or fewer were more likely associated with higher social service involvement in admissions. This result may be explained from a resource perspective. Smaller facilities are less likely to employ additional staff to handle admissions only work, and a team approach is likely used in the admissions process. Additionally, smaller facility size is linked to higher quality care (Harrington et al., 2000) as measured by fewer quality of care and quality of life deficiencies.

Geographical area was determined to be relational to higher SS involvement in admissions with nursing home located in non-metropolitan areas more likely to have higher social service involvement in admissions. In non-metropolitan areas, it is more likely that a team approach is used to carry out clinical tasks and every member of the clinical team is used to provide care to residents (Canada et al., 2020; Galambos, 2021). Social services as part of this integral team, would be used to assist in the admissions process.

In terms of social service involvement and CT, our results indicate a higher involvement of social services in CT for nursing homes with stand-alone SS departments. The presence of a stand-alone department is a concrete and visible means to demonstrate the value and importance of SS involvement in the clinical operations of the nursing home. This type of structure demonstrates organizational support for social services and the higher visibility is likely to be a factor in the increased involvement in CT.

Relational factors

In relational theory, influence results from relationships between workers, coworkers, and managers. First, it is important that relationships and communication exist within these working groups to provide an opportunity for dialogue and exchange of ideas. Second, the existence of such relationships has the potential to influence organizational culture, including norms, standards, and focal activities. Key relationships have the potential to define what is considered meaningful activities and practices. For influence to occur, relationships and communication between entities must exist (Hosking et al., 2013).

In the context of this study, relational factors were associated with the broader category of CT. Relationships with other professionals and family made a difference in terms of the level of involvement in CT. Specifically, nursing homes in which the SS director reported that their administrator regularly engaged the expertise of the SS department was associated with higher involvement in CT. Given that the nursing home administrator is ultimately in charge of the delegation of responsibility, this finding points to the importance of building strong relationships between social services and administration. Taking the time to educate the administrator on key CT tasks that can be assumed by SS departments will help to ensure strong involvement in this area. It is also important to train social workers new to working in nursing homes, communication skills that will reinforce positive relationships between the administrator and the SS department. R.P Bonifas (2011) study of nursing homes in Washington State also reinforces the importance of social service/administrator relationships. In the 2011 study, social service personnel supervised by their administrator reported higher levels of support.

SS directors who reported regular engagement with family members were also associated with higher involvement in CT. This finding is not surprising since several key tasks in CT require strong communication with family members. A strong factor in successful CT is to bring family members and significant others into the CT discussions early and frequently, particularly if family members will be providing support and assistance in these processes (Popejoy et al., 2020). SS departments should be trained in effective models of family work and communication to insure optimal involvement in care planning and transitions.

Another relational factor that proved significant was the perception that social workers had about their coworkers valuing the role of social services in resident and family work. Those directors who reported that their coworkers did not value the role of social services were associated with lower involvement in CT. Relationships with coworkers are key and the need to develop strong relationships with coworkers may help to improve involvement in CT activities. Indeed, R. P. Bonifas (2015) identified the importance of collaborative relationships in addressing the core needs of residents. Training on how to work within interdisciplinary teams and interdisciplinary team buildings may help strengthen coworker relationships.

The final relational factor associated with lower involvement in CT were identified barriers to strong psychosocial care. SS directors who reported low social service representation on key committees, not enough social service staff for number of residents, and lower emphasis on social and emotional over medical and nursing needs were associated with lower involvement in CT. Given the key role that social workers and SS play in attending to psychosocial needs of residents, it follows that nursing homes with a workplace culture that does not hold psychosocial needs in the same regard as medical needs would be associated with lower social service involvement in CT. Building a culture in the nursing home that values a holistic approach to care (Fields et al., 2012) may help to lessen these barriers. We can speculate that improving relationships with coworkers and providing education facility-wide about the benefits of psychosocial care may help to reduce some of these self-identified barriers.

Qualifications

Results indicate that nursing homes with SS directors with a social work degree (bachelor's or master's) or a master's degree in any field is associated with lower SS involvement in admissions processes. We speculate that this outcome may be a result of the master's-prepared social workers and SS staff being more involved in the psychosocial and managerial aspects of nursing home operations while SS staff without master's degrees may be used more directly in the admissions process to facilitate these admissions. Indeed, in Author's 2013 study of core functions of SS departments, psychosocial care functions such as providing emotional support to families and residents, handling disagreements, discussing advance directives, and working with residents with behavioral health issues were cited more frequently as tasks SS departments engage in over completion of admissions paperwork and orientation to the facility. Additionally, Roberts et al.'s (2020) finding that social service staff with higher qualifications are integral to improving behavioral symptoms and reducing antipsychotic medications and Bonifas (2015) finding that social workers routinely intervene in resident-to-resident aggression, supports the use of more qualified social service workers in complex care situations. This speculation is also supported by the research findings of Sussman and Dupuis (2014) who advocate for the use of social workers to attend to complex social service needs of residents.

Limitations

The limitations to this study are that there were several categorical variables that justified a logistic regression analysis. The use of this statistical method produced the results reported in this study. Another type of analysis may produce different results. Additionally, if there were more continuous variables, the results may also be reported differently. However, applying the logistic regression analysis produced important findings that will add to the professional literature. Additionally, the sample was of significant size with national representation to add strength to the present analysis.

Conclusions

This logistic regression reports on social service involvement in nursing homes within the processes of admissions and CT. Several structural factors such as amount of FTE to beds, ownership and independent status, geographical area, and size of facility were associated with higher admissions involvement and stand-alone departments linked to higher involvement in CT Relational factors such as engagement with nursing home administrator and engagement with family were associated with higher involvement with CT. Perceived devaluing of the psycho-social function by coworkers and barriers to providing psychosocial care were associated with lower involvement in CT. Recommendations include promoting structural and relational factors that support higher involvement of social services in CT, the development of training programs on interdisciplinary communication and team building skills, and the education of key staff to the role of social services in resident care. Finally, the development of an organizational culture that promotes a holistic, person-centered approach to care and supports the inclusion of psychosocial support is important to improve social service and social work involvement in care transitions.

ORCID

Mercedes Bern-Klug ⓘ http://orcid.org/0000-0001-6546-6141

References

Altfeld, S. J., Shier, G. E., Rooney, M., Johnson, T. J., Golden, R. L., & Perry, A. J. (2013). Effects of an enhanced discharge planning intervention for hospitalized older adults: A randomized trial. *The Gerontologist*, *53*(3), 430–440. https://doi.org/10.1093/geront/gns109

Alvarez, R., Ginsburg, J., Grabowski, J., Post, S., & Rosenberg, W. (2016). The Social Work Role in Reducing 30-Day Readmissions: The Effectiveness of the Bridge Model of Transitional Care. *Journal of Gerontological Social Work*, *59*(3), 222–227. https://doi.org/10.1080/01634372.2016.1195781

Auerbach, C., Mason, S. E., & Heft Laporte, H. (2007). Evidence that supports the value of social work in hospitals. *Social work in Health Care*, *44*(4), 17–32. https://doi.org/10.1300/J010v44n04_02

Bern-Klug, M., Mason, & Kramer, K. W. (2013). Core functions of nursing home social services departments in the United States. *Journal of the AmericanMedical Directors Association*, *14*(1), 75–e1–75–e7.

Bern -Klug, M., Smith, K.M., Roberts, A.R., Kusmaul, N., Gammonley, D., Hector, P., Simons, K., Galambos, C., Bonifas, R., Herman, C., Downes, D., Munn, J.C., Rudderham, G., Cores, E., Connolly, R. (2021). About a thirdof nursing home social services directors have earned a social work degree and license. *Journal of Gerontological Social Work*. doi: 10.1080/01634372.2021.1891594

Barber, R. D., Coulourides Kogan, A., Riffenburgh, A., & Enguidanos, S. (2015). A role for social workers in improving care setting transitions: A case study. *Social work in health care*, *54*(3), 177–192. https://doi.org/10.1080/00981389.2015.1005273

Berne Klug, M., & Beaulieu, E. (2020). COVID-19 highlights the need for trained social workers in nursing homes. *Journal of the American Medical Director's Association*, *21*(2020), 970e972. doi:10.1016/j.jamda.2020.05.049

Bonifas, R. (2008). Nursing home work environment characteristics: Associated outcomes in psychosocial care. *Health Care Financing Review*, *30*(2), 19–32. https://www.ncbi.nlm.nih.gov/pmc/articles/PMC4195053/

Bonifas, R. P. (2011). Multilevel Factors Related to Psychosocial Care Outcomes in Washington State Skilled Nursing Facilities. *Journal of Gerontological Social Work*, *54*(2), 203–223. https://doi.org/10.1080/01634372.2010.538817

Bonifas, R. P. (2015). Resident-to-resident aggression in nursing homes: Social worker involvement and collaboration with nursing colleagues. *Health & Social Work*, *40*(3), 101–109. https://doi.org/10.1093/hsw/hlv040

Bronstein, L., Gould, P., Berkowitz, S. A., James, G. D., & Marks, K. (2015). Impact of a Social Work Care Coordination Intervention on Hospital Readmission: A Randomized Controlled Trial. *Social Work*, *60*(3), 248–255. https://doi.org/10.1093/sw/swv016

Canada, K. E., Galambos, C., Pritchett, A., Rollin, L., Rantz, M., Popejoy, L., & Vogelsmeier, A. (2020). Transitions of care: Perspectives of patients living in long term care. Journal of Nursing Care Quality, 35(3), 189-94.

Code of Federal Regulations. (1987). Title 42: Public Health, Part 483, subpart b. Requirements for long term care facilities, section 483.15: Quality of life. Washington, D.C.: Government Printing Office.

Code of Federal Regulations. (1987). Title 42: Public Health, Part 483, subpart b. Requirements for long term care facilities, section 483.15: Quality of life. Washington, D.C.: Government Printing Office.

Fabbre, V. D., Buffington, A., Altfeld, S. J., Shier, G. E., & Golden, R. L. (2011). Social work and transitions of care: Observations from an intervention for older adults. *Journal of Gerontological Social Work*, *54*(6), 615–626. https://doi.org/10.1080/01634372.2011.589100

Fields, N. L., Koenig, T., & Dabelko-Schoeny, H. (2012). Resident transitions to assisted living: A role for social workers. *Health & social work*, *37*(3), 147. https://doi.org/10.1093/hsw/hls020

Fitzpatrick, J., & Tzouvara, V. (2019). Facilitators and inhibitors of transition for older people who have relocated to a long term care facility: A systematic review. *Health & social care in the community*, *27*(3), e57–e81. https://doi.org/10.1111/hsc.12647

Golden, R. L. (2011). Coordination, integration, and collaboration: A clear path for social work in health care reform. *Health & social work*, *36*(3), 227–228. https://doi.org/10.1093/hsw/36.3.227

Gruneir, A., Bronskill, S. E., Bell, C. M., Gill, S. S., Schull, M. J., Ma, X., & Rochon, P. A. (2012). Recent health care transitions and emergency department use by chronic long term care residents: A population-based cohort study. *Journal of the American Medical Directors Association*, *13*(3), 202–206. https://doi.org/10.1016/j.jamda.2011.10.001

Galambos, C. (2021). Social Work. In Kaye, L. (Ed). The handbook of rural aging.Philadelphia: Routledge, Taylor, and Francis. *Journal of Nursing Care Quality*, 35(3), 189–94.

Harrington, C., Woolhandler, S., Mullan, J., Carrillo, H., & Himmelstein, D. U. (2001). Does investor ownership of nursing homes compromise the quality of care? *American Journal of Public Health*, *91*(9), 1452–1455. https://doi.org/10.2105/AJPH.91.9.1452

Harrington, C., Zimmerman, D., Karon, S. L., Robinson, J., & Beutel, P. (2000). Nursing Home Staffing and Its Relationship to Deficiencies. *The Journals of Gerontology: Series B*, *55*(5), S278–S287. https://doi.org/10.1093/geronb/55.5.S278

Haveman, H. A., & Wetts, R. (2019). Organizational theory: From classical sociology to the 1970's. *Sociology Compass*, *13*(3), e12627. https://doi.org/10.1111/soc4.12627.

Holliman, D., Dziegielewski, S. F., & Teare, R. (2003). Differences and similarities between social work and nurse discharge planners. *Health & social work*, *28*(3), 224–231. https://doi.org/10.1093/hsw/28.3.224

Hosking, D. M., Dachler, H. P., & Gergen, K. J. (Eds). (2013). *Management and Organization: Relational Alternatives to Individualism*. Taos Institute Publications.

Jencks, S. F., Williams, M. V., & Coleman, E. (2009). Rehospitalizations among patients in the Medicare fee-for-service program. *The New England Journal of Medicine*, *360*(14), 1418–1428. https://doi.org/10.1056/NEJMsa0803563

Lipani, M., Holster, K., & Bussey, S.R. (2015). The preventable admissions care team (PACT): A social work -led Model of transitional care. *Social Work in Health Care54*(9), 810–827.

Lipani, M. B., Holster, K., & Bussey, S. R. (2015). The Preventable Admissions Care Team (PACT): A Social Work-Led Model of Transitional Care. *Social Work in Health Care*, *54*(9), 810–827. https://doi.org/10.1080/00981389.2015.1084970

NASW. (1981). *NASW Standards for Social Work Services in Long Term Care*.

NASW. (2003). *NASW Standards for Social Work Services in Long Term Care Facilities.*

O'Neill, C., Harrington, C., Kitchener, M., & Saliba, D. (2003). Quality of Care in Nursing Homes: An Analysis of Relationships among Profit, Quality, and Ownership. *Medical Care, 41*(12), 1318–1330. https://doi.org/10.1097/01.MLR.0000100586.33970.58

Popejoy, L. L., Vogelsmeier, A. A., Wakefield, B. J., Galambos, C. M., Lewis, A. M., Huneke, D., & Mehr, D. R. (2020). Adapting project RED to skilled nursing facilities. *Clinical Nursing Research, 29*(3), 149-156. https://doi.org/10.1177/1054773818819261

Roberts, A. R., Smith, A. C., & Bowblis, J. R. (2020). Nursing home social services and post acute care: Does more qualified staff improve behavioral symptoms and reduce antipsychotic drug use? *Journal of the American Medical Director's Association, 21*(3), 388–394. https://doi.org/10.1016/j.jamda2019.07.024

Simons, K., Bern-Klug, M., & An, S. (2012). Envisioning Quality Psychosocial Care in Nursing Homes: The Role of Social Work. *Journal of the American Medical Directors Association, 13*(9), 800–805. https://doi.org/10.1016/j.jamda.2012.07.016

Sims-Gould, J., Byrne, K., Hicks, E., Franke, T., & Stolee, P. (2015). "When Things Are Really Complicated, We Call the Social Worker": Post-hip-fracture care transitions for older people. *Health & social work, 40*(4), 257–265. https://doi.org/10.1093/hsw/hlv069

Smith, R. L., Ashok, M., & Morss, D. S. (2014). *Contextual Frameworks for Research on the Implementation of Complex System Interventions [Internet].* Agency for Healthcare Research and Quality (US). https://www.ncbi.nlm.nih.gov/books/NBK196206/

Sussman, T., & Dupuis, S. (2014). Supporting residents moving into long-term care: Multiple layers shape residents' experiences. *Journal of Gerontological Social Work, 57*(5), 438–459. https://doi.org/10.1080/01634372.2013.875971

Vourlekis, B. S., Bakke-Friedland, K., & Zlotnik, J. L. (1992). Clinical indicators to assess the quality of social work services in nursing homes. *Social Work in Health Care, 22*(1), 81–93. https://doi.org/10.1300/J010v22n01_06

Weerahandi, H., Basso Lipani, M., Kalman, J., Sosunov, E., Colgan, C., Bernstein, S., … Egorova, N. (2015). Effects of a Psychosocial Transitional Care Model on Hospitalizations and Cost of Care for High Utilizers. *Social Work in Health Care, 54*(6), 485–498. https://doi.org/10.1080/00981389.2015.1040141

Zhang, N. J., Gammonley, D., Paek, S. C., & Frahm, K. (2008). Facility service environments, staffing, and psychosocial care in nursing homes. *Health Care Financing Review, 30*(2), 5–17. https://pubmed.ncbi.nlm.nih.gov/19361113/

Zúñiga, F., Ausserhofer, D., Hamers, J. P., Engberg, S., Simon, M., & Schwendimann, R. (2015). The relationship of staffing and work environment with implicit rationing of nursing care in Swiss nursing homes–a cross-sectional study. *International Journal of Nursing Studies, 52*(9), 1463–1474. https://doi.org/10.1016/j.ijnurstu.2015.05.005

Dementia Tops Training Needs of Nursing Home Social Services Directors; Discharge Responsibilities Are Common Core Functions of the Department

Mercedes Bern-Klug ⓘD and Elizabeth Cordes

ABSTRACT

This report address two key questions: what are common core functions of nursing home social services departments and what are top training needs. Cross-sectional survey data collected in 2019 from a nationally representative sample of 924 social services directors reveal 33 responsibilities that at least two-thirds of respondents reported their department was usually or always involved in. We document strong and consistent interest in more training related to dementia and in common mental health and psychosocial challenges residents face. Findings reveal that training specific to social services is difficult to find. Online training opportunities were endorsed and 96% felt training targeted to new social services directors would be useful.

The purpose of this report is to describe the training needs of nursing home social services staff members. It is important to identify these training needs and to develop and disseminate training so that staff is prepared to provide the highest level of care, particularly, psychosocial care, to residents. In addition to providing care to residents, nursing home social services departments provide services to residents' families, including teaching coping skills, assisting with mental health referrals, coordinating discharge plans, providing case management services, and advocacy (Simons et al., 2012).

A literature review failed to identify a national study of social services training needs or any state-specific training need studies. There is no national organization exclusively focused on training needs of nursing home social services staff, although a few states, including Minnesota, Illinois, and Iowa, have voluntary statewide long-term care social worker organizations that provide training and support to members employed in nursing homes.

Nursing home trade organizations provide some training to social services staff who are employed by nursing homes that hold membership in the trade organization. These trainings are often targeted at all staff and less likely to be geared toward the unique role of social services. The National Association of Social Workers' (NASW) membership includes social workers employed in nursing homes, but the vast majority of its 120,000 members are not employed in nursing homes. NASW does provide training in geriatrics, palliative care, and end-of-life care as well as psychosocial care concerns for people with chronic illness; however, most of the training is not focused on the unique circumstances facing nursing home residents.

Social services staffing

In the case of Medicare and/or Medicaid certified nursing homes, the federal government requires only nursing homes with more than 120 beds to employ one full-time equivalent social services staff member. That staff member can hold a degree in social work (i.e., a professional social worker) or can hold a degree in a different field (including fields that do not require any clinical skills) (Code of Federal Regulations, 2020). Nursing homes with 120 or fewer beds are not required by federal regulations to employ any social services staff, and if they do, the staff can have any qualifications, including a high school degree. In this article, we refer to the department as the "social services department" and the director of the department as the "social services director." If the social services staff member is a person with a degree in social work, we call that person a "social worker." For more information about social services staffing in nursing homes please refer to Bern-Klug, Carter et al. (2021).

NASW has put forth professional standards for social work services in long-term care settings, including in nursing homes. The standards call for nursing home social workers to have at a minimum an undergraduate degree in social work from a program accredited by the Council on Social Work Education and a preference for the director of social services to have earned a master's degree in social work (NASW, 2003). With the CMS allowing high school graduates to lead social services department (in facilities with 120 or fewer beds) and the NASW calling for MSW prepared social workers as departmental directors, we expect broad variation in the functioning of social service departments throughout the country. That is why, as part of this study on training needs, we also report the responsibilities of social services departments throughout the country. It is important to understand the responsibilities of nursing home social services departments so that effective and efficient training can be developed and disseminated. Well-prepared social services staff are better able to meet the needs of residents, families, and fellow staff members.

The report has three objectives: to describe the most common responsibilities performed by nursing home social services departments in the US; to describe training needs as reported by social services directors; and to report the level of training support provided by nursing homes to their social services department.

Methods

These findings come from the *2019 National Nursing Home Social Services Directors Study*, administered by researchers at the University of Iowa School of Social Work, with support from the RRF Foundation for Aging.

Sample

The sample of nursing home social services directors represents 924 nursing homes in the United States. The sampling frame was the CMS publicly available data file from the Nursing Home Compare website. The random sample function in SPSS version 26 was used to draw a sample of 3,650 of the 15,578 Medicare and/or Medicaid certified nursing homes in December 2018. Because we did not know which of the nursing homes employed a social services staff person (our target respondent), each selected facility was telephoned to determine if at least one person was employed at least part-time in social services. If so, we asked for that person's name and e-mail address, so we could send an invitation to participate in the study. All told, 3067 invitations to participate in the study were emailed or ground mailed (if we did not receive a response from the e-mail invitation). We received 924 responses for a response rate of 30%. (For more details, refer to Bern-Klug, Smith et al., 2021.)

Survey instrument

The survey instrument contained 185 items including five open-ended questions. Respondents were asked about the role and responsibilities of the social services department, training interests, training supports available, departmental staffing, and whether the social services director felt prepared to train a new staff member in a series of tasks and processes.

Social services responsibilities

Two sets of questions collected information on social services responsibilities. Respondents were asked to indicate which sections of the Minimum Data Set (MDS) (resident assessment tool required by CMS in all certified nursing homes) were typically completed by the social services department. A second set of 46 questions asked respondents to indicate the extent to which the social services department was involved in activities such as screening for anxiety, coordinating admissions paperwork, or responding to family grievances. Possible answers included: social services is never involved, sometimes involved, usually involved, always involved, or "this is not done at our facility." The list of 46 tasks was inspired by the social work job description used in the VA system and NASW Standards for Long-term Care Services (NASW, 2003), and was finalized after vetting with 13 national advisors, all of whom had worked in nursing home social services or had been involved in nursing home research (see acknowledgments for list of advisors).

Training interest

Respondents were asked about their training interests and training needs in three different ways. First, we asked respondents to indicate their level of interest in 15 specific areas of training including psychosocial needs of persons with dementia and trauma-informed care. The question stem was "Social services staff work with other staff members to improve care. How interested are YOU in receiving training on how you can explain and support other staff with ... ." Possible responses were no interest, minor interest, moderate interest, strong interest. The second way training needs were measured was by directly asking respondents to indicate their top training priority. Respondents were asked to write in their response.

Proxy measure of training needs

Because our pilot testing indicated that many respondents would report interest in all areas of training, in order to help prioritize training needs, we developed another way of estimating them. In this third approach, we assessed training needs were less direct than the other two. We developed a set of 27 questions using this stem: "Please estimate how much preparation time you would need to provide one-on-one training to a social services colleague, about how to ... ." Examples included assessing pain; comparing/contrasting dementia, depression, and delirium; and assessing suicide risk. Possible responses included: could do without prep time, would need up to 2 hours of prep time, would need up to 10 hours of prep time, not able to do so. We combined "would need up to 10 hours" with "not able to do" as a proxy indication of training needs. We recognize that the ability to train one other person is not the exact same concept as needing to train oneself; however, as the director of social services, the respondent is expected to be able to train a colleague in certain areas related to social services. Not all respondents were expected to be able to train in all areas. The list of 27 items was approved by the 13-member national advisory committee.

Resident characteristics

The survey instrument contained two questions about the characteristics of residents in the nursing home. "About what percent of your nursing home residents have a serious mental illness such as schizophrenia, bi-polar disease, severe depression, or severe PTSD? (an estimate is Ok)" Possible answers included: Less than 10% of residents, 10–24%, 25–49%, 50% or more, and "I have no idea." The second question about residents was, "About what percent of social services staff time is spent on short-term patients (post-acute, sub-acute, rehab, skilled)? A rough estimate is OK." The answers were 0% percent of time, 1–24%, 25–49%, 50–74%, 75–99%, and 100%.

Employer support of continuing education

The survey asked respondents about training support in terms of continuing education available from their employer, using this question: "What level of continuing educational does your employer pay for or provide to you? (check ALL that apply)" with the possible answers: on-site training, permission to attend free training outside of work, will pay conference registration fee for an in-town conference, will pay conference registration fee, transportation and hotel for a conference out-of-town, my employer does not provide or pay for any continuing education for me.

Other training-related items

Questions about the difficulty in finding continuing education training specific to nursing home social services and interest in online education and a credential were also asked.

Analysis and human subjects

Univariate findings are represented in percentages. The University of Iowa's Institutional Review Board approved the study.

Findings

As reported in more detail elsewhere (Bern-Klug, Smith et al., 2021) the characteristics of the nursing homes that responded were similar to the national population of nursing homes, although nursing homes from the Midwest region were slightly over-represented.

Table 1. Characteristics of a nationally representative sample of 924 nursing home social services directors: 2019.

	Percent of 924 respondents
Women	92%
Race	
African American	6
White	88
Age-group	
18–25	4
26–34	24
35–44	24
45–54	23
55–64	19
65+	5
Highest Education	
High School	10
Associates Degree	6
Bachelors (non-SW)	20
Bachelors (SW)	**30**
Masters (non-SW)	7
Masters (SW)	**28**
SW Licensed or Certified	47
Completed an internship, practicum or field placement in a nursing home as part of formal education	30
Years of NH Social Services Experience:	
Less than 1	7
1–3 years	19
4–9 years	27
10–15 years	16
More than 15 years	31

Social services directors' characteristics

Table 1 reports characteristics of a nationally representative sample of nursing home social services directors. Over 90% were women, 88% reported their race as white, and 24% were aged 55 or older in 2019. Educational attainment ranged from a high school degree to a master's degree, with 58% of the sample having earned a bachelor's or master's degree in social work. Thirty percent of respondents completed an internship in a nursing home as part of their education and 26% had been in the job 3 years or less.

Social services department characteristics

Table 2 provides information about the characteristics of the social services department. In over half (54%) of nursing homes, there is only one person working in social services, in 31% there are two people working either full or part-time. Only 6% of nursing homes employed four or more social services staff members. Twenty percent of the respondents worked in nursing homes with fewer than 60 beds, 53% in facilities with 60–120, and 27% worked in nursing homes with more than 120 beds (data not shown). Providing evidence of the acuity of resident needs, over half of respondents indicated that over half

Table 2. Characteristics of the social services departments.

	Percent of 924 respondents
Number of employees in social services department:	
One person	54%
Two people	31
Three people	9
Four or more	6
Social services director's boss is the administrator	93
Social services is its own department	92
Nursing home has a contract with outside social services consultant who provides support and/or supervision to social services staff members	29
Percent of social services staff time spent on short-term patients (post-acute, sub-acute, rehab, or skilled)?	
0 time	2
1–24% of time	15
25–49% of time	25
50–74% of time	34
75–99% of time	18
100% of time	2
Percent of nursing home residents with a serious mental illness such as schizophrenia, bi-polar disorder, severe depression, or severe PTSD?	
Less than 10% of residents	40
10–24% of residents	28
25–49% of residents	18
50% or more	13

of social services efforts are devoted to post-acute residents and 31% of respondents indicated that at least 25% of residents in their facility had a serious mental illness.

Social services responsibilities

Tables 3 and 4 provide information about the role of the social services department. Table 3 reports staff involvement in completing the resident assessment instrument, the minimum data set (MDS). Out of the ten MDS items listed in the survey, over 80% of respondents indicated that their department typically completed these four sections: mood (95%); resident participation in assessment and goal setting (91%); cognitive status (87%) and behaviors (83%).

Table 3. Social services staff and completion of the MDS* (n = 924).

Which MDS sections are typically completed by social services staff?	%
Section D – Mood	95
Section Q – Participation in assessment and goal setting	91
Section C – Cognitive	87
Section E – Behaviors	83
Section B – Hearing and Vision	28
Section A – Identification	19
Section F – Routines	7
Section G – Functional Status	1
Section GG – Abilities and Goals	1
None	1
"other" (not listed)	15

* = MDS is the Minimum Data Set, a resident assessment instrument.

Table 4. Core functions of social services departments in 924 nursing homes: 2019.

	"To what extent is social services involved?" Possible answers: never, sometimes, usually, always, or "this is not done at our facility."	Percent "Usually or Always" Involved
1	Discharge planning for long-stay residents	97
2	Discharge planning for post-acute residents	96
3	Community services arrangement for residents transferring out	96
4	Developing individual care plans addressing psychosocial needs	96
5	Mediate issues between residents	96
6	Meet residents/family to discuss discharge plans 4–7 prior to discharge	95
7	Identify long-stay residents who might be candidates to be discharged to the community with services	93
8	Facilitate care plan meetings (manage time, mediate disagreements, keep team on track)	93
9	Refer residents to a mental health professional for individual counseling	93
10	Respond to family grievances	93
11	Engage residents and families in advance care planning conversations and document in medical record	93
12	Facilitate "goals of care" conversations with residents/families	91
13	Serve on QAPI committee (quality assurance & performance improvement)	91
14	Conduct a comprehensive biopsychosocial assessment	91
15	As part of admissions process, discuss tentative discharge plans with resident and family	89
16	Screen for depression	89
17	Review advance directives with resident/family at least quarterly	89
18	Plan staff interventions to prevent or minimize aggressive behaviors	89
19	Coordinate search for lost possessions of residents	88
20	Help decide resident transfer to a psychiatric unit	87
21	Document residents' goals for community connections outside the nursing home	82
22	Participate in disaster response planning and drills	81
23	Create safety plan for residents at risk of suicide	80
24	Meet with resident/family to balance resident self-determination with NHs responsibility for safety; document	79
25	Document residents' goals for personal growth	78
26	Meet with resident/family on discharge day to discuss plans	77
27	Provide summary of care plan meeting to resident/family	77
28	Participate in developing level 2 PASARR care plans for residents with serious mental illness or intellectual disabilities	77
29	Screen residents for anxiety	75
30	Document residents' preferences for daily living	69
31	Recommend changes to organizational policies and procedures aimed at improving psychosocial care	67
32	Discuss POLST with residents/family [Physician Orders for Life-Sustaining Treatment]	67
33	Explain Title 19 (Medicaid) application process to resident/family	66
34	Explain what is and is not covered by different insurances (Medicare, Medicaid, VA)	62
35	Assist residents with technology challenges (cell phone, laptop, tablets, etc.)	57

(Continued)

Table 4. (Continued).

36	Participate in Process improvement Projects (PIPs)	57
37	Provide counseling (psychotherapy) sessions directly with residents who have depression and/or mood disorder	52
38	Conduct a follow-up call/visit to resident within 7 days of discharge	50
39	Coordinate the admissions paperwork	45
40	Review preadmission documentation to determine suitability for admission	42
41	Arrange transportation for resident to receive health care	30
42	Visit potential residents in hospital/home to assess for admission	19
43	Assist with delivering recreational activities	17
44	Screen for pain	16
45	Recruit, coordinate, supervise volunteers	9
46	Help feed residents at mealtime	9

Table 4 reports results from asking about social services departmental involvement in a series of 46 tasks. Two-thirds and more of respondents indicated the social services department was usually or always involved in 33 of the 46 tasks, with over 90% of respondents, indicating "usual or always" involvement in 14 tasks. At the top of the list was discharge planning for long-stay residents (97% of respondents) followed by discharge planning for short-stay residents (96%). Ninety-six percent of respondents also reported their department was usually or always involved with these tasks: community services arrangements for residents transferring out, developing individual care plans addressing psychosocial needs, and mediating issues between residents.

Employer support of continuing education

Table 5 summarizes responses regarding questions related to continuing education. While 60% reported their employer provided on-site training and 63% reported their employer would allow them to attend free training outside of work, 15% indicated their employer neither provides nor pays toward their continuing education. Over half (63%) of respondents reported it was difficult to find continuing education opportunities directly related to nursing home social services. The vast majority (91%) reported interest in online continuing education geared to social services, and 96% reported they thought it would be useful for new social services staff to participate in training that explains the nursing home context and core social services responsibilities.

Table 5. Responses from 924 nursing home social services directors regarding continuing education: 2019.

	Percent of 924 respondents
Level of continuing education provided or paid for by employer:	
Permission to attend free training outside of work	63
On-site training	60
Will pay conference registration fee for an in-town conference	47
Will pay conference registration fee, transportation, and hotel for out-of-town conference	36
Employer does not pay for or provide continuing education	15
Somewhat (51%) or very (12%) difficult to find continuing education opportunities directly related to nursing home social services	63
Somewhat (39%) or very (52%) interested in online continuing education geared toward nursing home social services directors	91
Somewhat (35%) or very (49%) interested in opportunity to earn a credential in "nursing home social services" for social services directors with at least 3 years of experience. (Includes completing 6–8 online modules (presentations, small-group online discussions) and an exam.)	84
Somewhat (25%) or very (71%) useful for new social services staff members to participate in 6–8, one-hour online training sessions explaining the nursing home context and core social services responsibility.	96

Table 6. Level of interest among 924 nursing home social services directors in receiving training on how to explain and support other staff with a variety of activities and processes.

"Social services staff work with other staff members to improve care. **How interested are YOU in receiving training on how you can explain and support other staff with:** *"*	Moderate or Strong Interest	Strong Interest	Minor Interest	No Interest
1　**... psychosocial needs of persons with dementia**	86%	59%	8%	5%
2　... common **mental health and psychosocial challenges** faced by residents	86	56	8	4
3　... **establishing trust** with a resident and/or family who feels mistreated by the nursing home or by a staff member	78	52	14	7
4　... improving staff relationships with family members of residents	78	50	14	6
5　... fostering a social environment (culture) where grievances are welcomed and seen as opportunities for improvement	78	48	14	7
6　**... resident rights**	76	48	14	8
7　... types of **resident abuse, neglect** and/or **exploitation by** staff, residents, family and/or other visitors	75	48	16	8
8　... interacting with visitors whose behaviors are perceived as threatening to residents or to staff	75	45	16	8
9　... understanding and supporting residents with addiction such as **alcohol, substances, gambling, gaming, and/or hoarding**	75	44	15	9
10　... **cultural humility and culturally competent care**	74	40	17	8
11　... **nonpharmacological approaches to addressing pain**	72	41	17	10
12　... **trauma-informed care**	70	42	17	12
13　... issues related to **expressions of intimacy and sexuality** (for cognitively intact and impaired residents)	65	37	24	10
14　... **discrimination** against residents, families, or staff on account of **age, disability, race, ethnicity, and/or religion**	65	36	23	11
15　... **discrimination** against residents, families, or staff on account of **sexual orientation** and/or **gender identity**	64	36	23	11

Training interests and needs

Table 6 reports the results from 15 questions that asked respondents to indicate their level of interest in receiving training. Close to two-thirds (64%) or more (up to 86%) reported moderate-to-strong interest in all 15 topics. With the highest percentage reporting interest in training related to the psychosocial needs of persons with dementia (86%), and training on common mental health and psychosocial challenges faced by residents (86%).

Amount of preparation time needed to train a colleague

Table 7 reports results from a series of 27 questions asking about the amount of preparation time the respondent would need to train a fellow social services staff member. Listed are two columns, the right column lists the percentage of respondents who indicated they would not need any prep time to train someone else and the left column reports the respondents who would need up to 10 hours of prep time (or not able to train a colleague). We consider people in the left column as candidates for needing training in those areas. There were 13 tasks in which at least 20% of respondents are candidates for training. The

Table 7. Social services directors' self-reported preparation time necessary to provide one-on-one training to a social services colleague: 2019, n = 924.

	Please estimate how much _preparation time_ you would need to provide one-on-one training to a social services colleague, about how to: (possible answers: could do without prep time; would need up to 2 hours prep time; would need up to 10 hours prep time; not able to do)	10+ hours or "not able to do"	Could do without prep time
1	... secure a **legal guardian** for a resident	38%	19%
2	... **assess pain** in residents (with or without dementia) and develop a care plan to address the psychosocial aspects of pain	36	24
3	... work with residents with **limited (or no) ability to speak** or read English	35	18
4	... teach **risk management and critical thinking skills**, including how the medical record can be used during a survey or court proceeding	34	19
5	... review the main **state and federal regulations** affecting the provision of social services in nursing homes	30	20
6	... discuss **common psychotropic drugs**, their uses, side effects (including mood/psychosocial), and the principle of gradual dose reduction	29	23
7	... explain health insurance benefits, VA benefits and common out-of-pocket expenses encountered by residents	28	25
8	... develop care plans for residents with **serious mental health concerns** including severe depression, schizophrenia, bi-polar disorder and/or PTSD	25	20
9	... assess and develop care plans to address the psychosocial needs of residents with **end-stage renal disease receiving kidney dialysis**	24	20
10	... compare/contrast **dementia, depression, and delirium** and anticipate common psychosocial needs	22	21
11	... work with residents who are **behaving aggressively** toward others	20	31
12	... assess **suicide risk** in residents who are depressed, develop (and carry out) a safety plan and provide appropriate documentation in the chart	20	30
13	... describe how the **nursing home is funded**, how social services contributes to resident quality of life and to the financial status of the nursing home	20	39
14	... assess psychosocial needs of **younger residents** (under age 60), develop care plan and connect with appropriate community resources	19	25
15	... conduct a comprehensive biopsychosocial assessment, develop and document measurable goals, and provide/oversee care	19	23
16	... conduct a **POLST conversation** with residents/families and complete the form, if applicable. POLST = Physician Orders for Life Sustaining Treatment also known as MOLST or IPOST	17	45
17	... anticipate and plan for common _psychosocial reasons_ for medically **unnecessary rehospitalizations**, and work with resident, family, and staff to avoid	17	29
18	... anticipate and plan for common _psychosocial reasons_ for medically unnecessary rehospitalizations **AFTER DISCHARGE HOME**, and work to address	17	33
19	... identify **ethical issues** and use an ethical framework to guide action	17	31
20	... work with resident/family and team to balance **resident self-determination** with the NH's responsibility to **minimize risk** (and chart the conversation)	14	33
21	... work with residents who are **experiencing grief and loss**	12	34
22	... incorporate residents' **strengths, preferences, values, and goals** into their care plan	11	35
23	... explain the **social services' role in disaster** planning and during a disaster	11	39
24	... describe the characteristics of residents who may benefit from **counseling services provided by a licensed mental health professional**, how to arrange the services, and explain how the services will be paid for	9	45
25	... discuss **advance directives options** (medical directives, living wills, and appointing a health care agent)	8	55
26	... engage residents/families in **advance care planning conversations**, including discussing palliative care and hospice options	8	52
27	... **request a "mental health consultation"** with a psychologist, clinical social worker, or other mental health professional	7	56

four areas in which at least one-third of respondents reported they could not train on or would need up to 10 hours of preparation time in order to train a social services colleague include how to secure a legal guardian for a resident (38% not able to do or would require up to 10 hours of prep time); pain assessment and care planning (36%); how to work with residents with limited (or no) ability to speak or read English (35%); and how to teach risk management and critical thinking skills, including how the medical record can be used during a survey or court proceeding (34%). Table 7 shows that although some social services directors would need up to 10 hours of preparation time or simply could not train a colleague, in all 27 topic areas, at least 18% and up to 56% of respondents indicated they did not need *any* preparation time to train a colleague on the topic.

Top training priority

Table 8 shows the responses to the question asking respondents to write in their top training priority. Most respondents (n = 626) did write in a priority. We grouped the responses into broad categories. Training on dementia was the most frequently reported priority (20% of write-in responses) followed by clarification on federal or state regulations (17%) and training related to behavioral health (12%).

The most common dementia-related training need, by far, was how to interrupt or deal with aggressive behaviors of residents with dementia. Examples of other dementia-related training topics included: psychosocial

Table 8. Training priority reported by 626 NH Social Services Directors.

	What is your highest training priority? (grouped responses to open-ended question)	Percent
1	Dementia (behavioral management, co-occurring depression, assessing capacity, working with family)	21%
2	Regulations (including Patient Driven Payment Model)	17
3	Behavioral Health	12
4	Trauma-Informed Care	9
5	Care Planning (documentation)	6
6	End of Life issues	5
7	Medications (drug abuse, psychotropic meds)	5
8	General Social Services Information	4
9	Ethics (e-communication, sexual expression)	4
10	Miscellaneous/Other	4
11	Discharge Planning	3
12	PASARR	3
13	Residents Rights	2
14	Abuse	2
15	Person-Centered Care	2
16	Cultural Competence	1

Other priority areas mentioned: medical marijuana, Medicaid planning, dental needs, brain research, compassion fatigue, dealing with residents who have substantial past recreation drug use, rehospitalizations, dealing with residents and/or families with a history of domestic abuse, working with "radical" families, managing overworked and overwhelmed fellow staff members, information technology, resources for people experiencing homelessness, and how to be a better supervisor.

care plans for people with dementia; depression and dementia; delirium; psychotropic medications and residents with dementia; and understanding the stages of dementia. Respondents who indicated regulations as a top training priority mentioned topics such as: Medicare payment for durable medical equipment, new F-tags for social services, keeping up with new federal regulations, knowing how to document to show compliance with regulations, and state survey paperwork requirements. Examples of behavioral health-related training priorities included: helping residents with mental health issues who are behaving aggressively toward other residents, assisting direct care staff with resident behavioral issues, and staff self-regulation dealing with residents with behavioral issues. It is possible that many of the respondents who simply wrote in "resident behaviors" were concerned about the behaviors of people with dementia.

Most of the 626 responses were training topics we had mentioned earlier in the survey; however, there were some new topics. The bottom of Table 8 includes some items not asked about earlier in the survey including medical marijuana, how to be a better supervisor, neurology and brain research updates, how to comfort family members after a resident dies, and resources for people experiencing homelessness.

Limitations

The 30% response rate is lower than we would like. Only social services directors were included in the study. Also, because of space, we limited the number of items listed as potential areas of social services involvement in the daily life of the nursing home and in possible training topics. Our lists are not exhaustive. Another limitation is using the "time needed to prepare a colleague" as a proxy measure for respondents' training needs.

Discussion

This report documents that nursing home social services departments are involved in a broad range of activities ranging from organizing the search for lost possessions to helping to create a safety plan for a resident at risk of attempting suicide. Our results indicate a core set of 29 activities that 75% of nursing home social services directors report their department is usually or always involved in, many of which are related to discharge planning, transitions of care, and psychosocial care planning. Departmental involvement with family members of residents also featured prominently among the common responsibilities of social services staff.

This is the first nationally representative study that reports on the training needs of nursing home social services staff members. Training related to providing care for residents with dementia was the dominant training need identified by social services directors. At least one-third of respondents indicated a strong interest in all 15 training topics we listed, with the highest being a tie between interest in the psychosocial needs of persons with dementia and interest in common mental health and psychosocial challenges faced by residents. When asked to write in their top training priority, dementia training was most frequently mentioned. While basic training about dementia is important for all staff members, social services staff members need to know how to assess and develop care plans that address the psychosocial needs of persons with dementia, work with residents whose behavior is troublesome to other residents, and update care plans to reflect resident wishes as expressed by the resident when able, or the family when the resident is no longer able to communicate. Social services directors sent a clear message that more training related to dementia is needed.

This study also asked respondents how much preparation time would be needed to train a colleague on 27 topics. We used this as a proxy measure for training needs. This question worked well to show the variation in the ability to train another social services colleague. For each of the 27 items, there were some respondents who reported they needed no prep time to train a colleague while other respondents reported they would need up to 10 hours or they could not train on that topic at all. The top four topics that social services directors expressed needing up to 10 hours (or not being able to do) were securing a legal guardian, pain and psychosocial implications for care planning, working with non-English speakers, and risk management.

The need for training related to pain is particularly important because of the high prevalence of pain among residents regardless of the region of the country or the size of the facility. Another justification for the need for more training on pain is that there can be serious psychosocial consequences of unaddressed pain (Linton & Shaw, 2011; Turk & Monarch, 2018). Reinforcing the need for pain-related training is our finding that only 16% of social services departments are "usually or always" involved with screening for pain. Clearly, there is room for far more social services involvement in helping to screen for pain and in developing care plans that address the psychosocial implications of pain, including among residents with dementia.

The findings indicate both a strong need and a strong desire among nursing home social services directors for more training specific to social services, and an openness to online training. A complication for people designing continuing education for nursing home social services staff is the broad range of educational preparedness found among staff ranging from a high school degree to a master's degree. It will be challenging to develop trainings that are useful and engaging to both educational extremes.

While we document a strong desire for additional training, it is important to note that federal regulations do not require continuing education for social services staff. That may be a reason why 15% of nursing homes do not provide or pay for continuing education for their social services staff. Staff who are licensed will need to pursue continuing education to remain licensed, but non-licensed personnel have no such requirements. As we report here, half of the directors of social services in the US nursing homes are not licensed or certified for social work.

Another contribution to the literature is the finding that almost one-third of social services directors completed an internship in a nursing home as part of their education. This finding underscores the importance of providing internship opportunities in nursing homes. More research is needed to determine aspects of an internship that promote student interest and commitment to this setting. We document strong interest in online continuing education and especially strong support for an online set of training modules for new social services staff members to learn about the nursing home context and the role of social services. Many (29%) of respondents reported having access to a social services consultant for support and professional supervision. Research is called for learning about the consultant role and the impact on the social services department of contracting with a social services consultant.

In summary, nursing home social service staff members are responsible for a broad range of processes and tasks that contribute to the daily life of the nursing home and that play an important role in the provision of psychosocial care to residents and support to families. If society expects social service staff to be able to provide excellent care to residents and families, staff need access to excellent training and support. We report areas of training needs and encourage NASW, trade associations, schools of social work, and state social work long-term care organizations to use these findings to craft training opportunities.

Acknowledgments

Special thanks to members of the Advisory Committee: Robin Bonifas, Bob Connolly, Deirdre Downes, Colleen Galambos, Denise Gammonley, Paige Hector, Chris Herman, Rosalie Kane, Nancy Kusmaul, Amy Lemke, Jean Munn, Amy Restorick Roberts, and Kelsey Simons.

Funding

This project was supported by the Iowa Geriatric Education Center and the Health Resources and Services Administration (HRSA) of the U.S. Department of Health and Human Services (HHS) under grant number U1QHP28731 the Geriatrics Workforce Enhancement Program. This information or content and conclusions are those of the author and should not be construed as the official position or policy of, nor should any endorsements be inferred by HRSA, HHS or the U.S. Government.

ORCID

Mercedes Bern-Klug ⓘ http://orcid.org/0000-0001-6546-6141

Conflict of interest

The authors have no conflicts to report.

References

Bern-Klug, M., Carter, K. A., & Wang, Y. (2021 under review). More evidence that federal regulations perpetuate unrealistic nursing home social services staffing ratios.

Bern-Klug, M., Smith, K. M., Roberts, A. R., Kusmaul, N., Gammonley, D., Hector, P., Simons, K., Galambos, C., Bonifas, R. P., Herman, C., Downes, D., Munn, J. C., Rudderham, G., Cordes, E., & Connolly, R. (2021). About a third of nursing home social services directors have earned a social work degree and license. *Journal of Gerontological Social Work*, 1–22. https://doi.org/10.1080/01634372.2021.1891594

Code of Federal Regulations. (2020). Title 42 (public health), chapter IV, subchapter G, part 483, subpart B (administration): https://www.ecfr.gov/cgi-bin/text-idx?SID=e7135feb0af73 c5ae7c97f690d995ae9&mc=true&node=se42.5.483_170&rgn=div8)

Linton, S. J., & Shaw, W. S. (2011). Impact of psychological factors in the experience of pain. *Physical Therapy*, *91*(5), 700–711. https://doi.org/10.2522/ptj.20100330

NASW. (2003). NASW standards for social work services in long-term care facilities. National Association of Social Workers. https://www.socialworkers.org/LinkClick.aspx?fileticket= cwW7lzBfYxg%3D&portalid=0

Simons, K., Connolly, R. P., Bonifas, R. P., Allen, P., Bailey, K., Downes, D., & Galambos, C. (2012). Psychosocial assessment of nursing home residents via MDS 3.0: Recommendations for social service training, staffing, and roles in interdisciplinary care. *Journal of the American Medical Directors Association*, *13*(2), 190.e9–190.e15. https://doi.org/10.1016/j. jamda.2011.07.005

Turk, D. C., & Monarch, E. S. (2018). Biopsychosocial perspectives on chronic pain. In D. C. Turk & R. J. Gatchel (Eds.), *Psychological approaches to pain management* (pp. 3–24).chapter 1 pages. Guilford Press.

Structural Characteristics of Nursing Homes and Social Service Directors that Influence Their Engagement in Disaster Preparedness Processes

Nancy Kusmaul ⓘ, Susanny Beltran, Tommy Buckley, Allison Gibson ⓘ, and Mercedes Bern-Klug ⓘ

ABSTRACT

Nursing home residents are an at-risk population during disaster situations, and nursing homes face unique challenges in managing disasters. Nursing home social service departments can support their nursing homes in meeting the needs of residents during disasters, yet there is little research exploring their involvement. To address this gap, we use secondary data from the 2019 National Nursing Home Social Service Directors' study to explore social service directors' and their departments' involvement in disaster preparedness and response, and personal- and nursing home-level characteristics that predict involvement. Results show that nursing home social service directors and their staffs are predominantly involved; 61.9% (n = 562) of respondents stated always participating, and an additional 20.3% (n = 184) usually participating in disaster planning. The age of the director significantly predicted involvement, with older directors being most likely to always be involved. Further research is needed to understand why some nursing homes involve their social service directors in disaster planning and others do not, what roles those directors play, and to identify strategies to increase involvement within this role.

Compared to older adults in the community, nursing home residents are at greater risk for adverse outcomes during disasters, in part due to older age and having more chronic conditions (Dosa et al., 2012). Nursing home residents often have functional limitations in activities of daily living (ADLs) and instrumental activities of daily living (IADLs), physical disabilities, and/or cognitive impairments that impact their ability to evacuate safely during disasters (Aldrich & Benson, 2008; Holup et al., 2017; Lu et al., 2020).

Nursing home social service departments "provide medically-related social services to attain or maintain the highest practicable physical, mental and psychosocial well-being of each resident" (Behavioral Health Services, 2016, para a). They also comprise essential parts of the interdisciplinary teams. Each nursing home approaches disaster preparedness differently, from what disciplines comprise the team to the role each plays in planning, practice/drills, and response (Office of Inspector General, 2012a). The Centers for Medicare and Medicaid Services (CMS) provides guidance in the form of a checklist (Emergency Preparedness Requirements for Medicare and Medicaid Participating Providers and Suppliers, 2016), which lays out what contingencies should be addressed in a nursing home's emergency plan but does not include which disciplines within the nursing home should be involved. Social services should be an important part of the plan, as the checklist calls for "Training ... to address psychological and emotional aspects on caregivers, families, residents, and the community at large" (Office of Inspector General, 2012b, p. 33). Other key elements of the regulation are procedures to assess for relevant hazards and developing interventions for each hazard; plans for communication with families, residents, transportation and other vendors; and instructions for policies and procedures to address the same.

Nursing homes face all types of hazards in disasters. While the CMS checklist does not designate which disciplines should be involved in disaster preparedness, the skills that bachelor's and master's prepared social workers bring to the long-term care environment, such as broker, advocate, manager, educator, facilitator, and organizer (e.g., Hepworth et al., 2013) could be particularly useful in helping nursing homes prepare for disasters. Nursing home social service directors, who may or may not be social workers, must understand micro, mezzo, and macro issues, be aware of person-in-environment, and have crisis management skills, all of which are essential components of social work education (Council on Social Work Education, 2015). Nursing homes with more qualified social service employees receive fewer psychosocial deficiencies on state inspection surveys (Simons, 2006).

Federal regulations require nursing homes with at least 120 beds that accept Medicare or Medicaid funds to have at least one full-time social worker, yet the definition of social worker includes people who are not educated or credentialed in social work. The regulatory definition of a social worker includes those with bachelor's degrees in gerontology, sociology, special education, rehabilitation counseling, and psychology (Administration, 2019). The National Association of Social Workers (NASW) recommends, at minimum, a nursing home social worker have a degree in social work (Bailey et al., 2003). We will discuss further in the literature review what makes social workers well suited to help in these activities.

Natural disasters are commonly defined by nursing home staff and researchers as events like hurricanes, tornadoes, and snowstorms, with the potential to physically damage buildings, disrupt the supply chain, and strand staff at work or away from the nursing home for extended periods of time (Goldman & Galea, 2014). This article uses data from the National Nursing

Home Social Services Directors' (NNHSSD) study, a nationally representative survey designed to characterize the nation's social services workforce, to describe the personal-level and nursing home-level structures that influence how often nursing home social service directors and their staffs are involved in the process of nursing home disaster preparedness. We also discuss the importance of including nursing home social service directors and workers in disaster preparedness and response and the strengths social workers can bring to these roles.

Literature Review

Nursing Homes and Disaster Preparedness and Response

With the exception of hospitals, nursing homes provide the highest level of care for older adults of any other setting. The frailty of this population decreases their ability to withstand negative situations that may occur before, during, and after disasters, such as gaps in care from personnel shortages, extreme changes in temperature, loss of necessary medical equipment due to power outages or floods, and sudden and unpredictable changes in setting or location, which can exacerbate confusion, agitation, and behavioral concerns (Brown et al., 2007; Fernandez et al., 2002).

The unique vulnerabilities of nursing home residents to disasters were highlighted during Hurricane Katrina in 2005, when approximately 139 nursing home residents died during and after the hurricane (Hyer et al., 2007). Subsequent studies exploring the morbidity and mortality impacts of being exposed to hurricanes indicate that the hurricane had long-term effects on nursing home residents (Dosa et al., 2010). Hurricane Katrina and its' ill effects revealed significant gaps in nursing homes' policies and planning and preparedness processes. A report issued by the Office of Inspector General (2006) indicated a breakdown had occurred in the planning process across all the Gulf States (Alabama, Florida, Louisiana, Mississippi, and Texas) that experienced a major hurricane in 2004 or 2005 (Ivan, Katrina, Rita, and Wilma). Factors contributing to breakdowns in preparedness and response included nursing homes not having adequate plans, administrators failing to follow through with planned processes, or plans not being sufficient to meet emerging needs during disasters. Nursing home administrators also reported that their exclusion from local, state, and federal planning efforts resulted in a lack of resources and supports during the disaster and that plans for older adults were inconsistent across the care continuum (Ladika et al., 2008).

The Potential Merits of Social Work in Disaster Planning and Response

Although social workers have often responded to disasters and traumas (Hamler et al., 2020; Kusmaul et al., 2018; Naturale, 2007; Scoville, 1942), there is a dearth of research specifically examining the role of social work in disaster response in nursing homes. Much of the existing literature discusses events that occurred over a decade ago, such as Hurricanes Katrina, Rita, and Gustav, or is conceptual (Beltran et al., 2020). These studies describe social work's role as supporting the emotional well-being of residents, and also that of overwhelmed, tired, and distressed direct care staff to ensure the team can function effectively under duress (Ladika et al., 2008). Social workers engage in disaster management activities throughout all stages of the disaster. For example, they provide individualized support to residents experiencing psychological distress from seeing news coverage about the impending events, restore communication with families (e.g., after evacuating to another location), and facilitate the processing of shared trauma (Claver et al., 2013; Ladika et al., 2008). As part of the interdisciplinary team, social workers are often the profession tasked with ensuring residents' emotional well-being. Nursing home administrators identify social work as the profession most likely to engage in resilience-building interventions such as psychological first aid training to support nursing home residents during disasters (Brown et al., 2010).

Other critical roles of nursing home social service workers are facilitating discussions about goals of care, resolving family conflicts, and documenting advance care planning wishes (Bomba et al., 2011). Ensuring resident goals are documented and up to date is crucial during disasters, as decisions may need to be made urgently or while communication with decision-makers is disrupted. Social workers collaborate with other members of the interdisciplinary team and outside agencies (e.g., hospice agencies), to plan for continuity of supports during disasters. Following a disaster, social workers support residents who have experienced a change in condition and their families; this may involve additional discussions around goals, and coordination of end-of-life care (Frahm et al., 2012).

Theoretical Framework

Donabedian's structure, process, and outcome model (Donabedian, 1988) for evaluating the quality of care is used as a framework to organize this exploratory study. Donabedian proposed that favorable client outcomes, or good quality care, results from effective processes, which are shaped by structural factors. Structures of healthcare include provider and organizational-level characteristics such as capacity (i.e., bed size, staffing); processes include how and what services are delivered; and outcomes are care quality and patient physical and psychosocial well-being. As described in the literature review, previous studies have highlighted the poor quality of disaster response in nursing homes, which is the Donabedian outcome of focus in our research. In this exploratory study, we focus on the role of facility-level and social service director-level characteristics (structure) on involvement in disaster preparedness (process).

Despite the potential for nursing home social service directors to engage in disaster preparedness and response, their level of involvement in this work within nursing homes has not been clearly described (Beltran et al., 2020). There are even fewer studies that speak directly to nursing home social service directors' and staffs' involvement in disaster preparedness. The current study helps to bridge this gap, by exploring nursing home social service directors' involvement in the process of disaster planning and response and the structural factors associated with that involvement.

Methods

Data Source

We used a subset of the NNHSSD study to describe whether nursing home social service workers help their nursing homes prepare for disasters and the personal-level and nursing home-level characteristics that influence that involvement. The NNHSSD study provides nationally representative data from nursing home social service directors to characterize the nation's nursing home social services workforce, describe their workload, and determine their training needs and preferences (Bern-Klug et al., 2021). The total survey had 185 items.

Of the 3,067 nursing home social service directors contacted by the NNHSSD study, 924 completed the study survey, for a response rate of 30%. The distribution of responses in the overall sample is reported in (Bern-Klug et al., 2021). Importantly, the nursing home characteristics of the respondents were representative of nursing homes nationally across multiple factors including the type of nursing home, ownership, bed size, chain status, and quality rating (Bern-Klug et al., 2021).

Variables

Outcome Variables

The primary outcomes we used are based on two items. The first item asked social service directors the extent to which social services staff "participate in disaster response planning and drills." Possible responses were "always", "usually", "sometimes", and "never". In our analysis, we combined sometimes and never due to the size of the samples, 12 ($n = 109$) and six ($n = 56$) percent, respectively, much smaller than the usually and always groups. The second item asked social service directors how much preparation time they would need in order to provide one-on-one training to a social services colleague to "explain the social services' role in disaster planning and during a disaster." Response options were "could do without preparation", "2 hours prep time", "10 hours prep time", or "could not do." This variable, particularly the "could not do" response, served as a proxy for whether or not they needed training themselves.

Predictor Variables

Predictor variables were selected to allow us to explore structural factors that might influence whether or not social service directors were involved in the disaster preparedness planning process. Due to the exploratory nature of this work, variables included were selected based on previous literature indicating their influence on nursing home processes and outcomes (e.g., Castle & Ferguson, 2010; Schnelle et al., 2004). We grouped the structural variables into individual-level factors and nursing home-level factors. Individual-level factors were education level, years of experience, whether the person had a social work degree and license or not, gender, race, and age. Demographic characteristics allow us to describe the sample. Other individual characteristics were based on the literature and NASW recommendations describing desired structural qualifications of social service staffing. To reduce respondent burden, nursing home-level factors were obtained from public access files on the CMS website. Nursing home-level variables were bed size, staffing ratio, ownership, location, and rural/urban designation. These structural variables have been shown in previous research to impact outcomes for nursing home residents (Shippee et al., 2015).

Individual Variables. The NNHSSD study collected information on social service directors and their staffs, as reported by the directors. We used information only about the directors themselves. Individual-level variables were kept as the NNHSSD study coded them. Education level was coded into three categories: less than a four-year degree, Bachelor's degree, and Master's degree. Years of experience was coded into three categories: 0–3 years, 4–9 years, and 10 or more years. Social work degree and license were coded as to whether the respondent had both a social work degree and a social work license (yes or no). Gender was coded as male and female. Race was coded into two categories: White and nonwhite, given the high percentage of White respondents (88.0%) in this sample. Age was collected as categorical, into ages 18–34, 35–54, and 55 and older.

Bed Size. Bed size refers to the number of Medicare and/or Medicaid certified beds. The NNHSSD study collapsed this into a categorical variable of 0–60, 61–120, and 120 + . These cut points reflect two structural factors. The average size of a nursing home in the United States is 106 beds; only one state has an average of fewer than 60 beds (Kaiser Family Foundation, 2019). Therefore, the 0–60 bed category was created to capture staffing differences that may occur in smaller homes. The cut point at 120 was due to the regulations that require a "full-time qualified social worker" in nursing homes with more than 120 beds (Administration, 2019).

Staffing Ratio. We calculated staffing ratio by dividing number of full-time equivalent social service staff by number of residents in the nursing home and then multiplying by 100.

Ownership. The CMS website lists 13 categories of tax status. For the NNHSSD study, these were collapsed into "for-profit", "not-for-profit", and "government."

Location. Researchers from the NNHSSD study obtained state level data on each nursing home and included it in the data set. Since this study looked at disaster preparedness, we collapsed the states into categories described as "Northeast Coastal" (mid-Atlantic and north), "South Coastal" (Gulf coast and southeastern U.S.), "West Coastal" (states that border on the Pacific Ocean), and "non-coastal" (all other states that do not border an ocean). We based these categories on the different types of potential disasters each was most likely to face, which we hypothesized would lead to differences in preparedness. We later re-categorized these into a new variable to examine differences in "Wildfire" versus "non-Wildfire" regions. The Wildfire category included Oregon, Washington, California, and Colorado, and non-Wildfire included the remaining states.

Rural/Urban. The NHHSSD study used county-level data to assign one of nine Rural-Urban continuum codes (RUCC) as designated by the USDA to each participating nursing home. For our analysis, the nine RUCC categories were collapsed into a dichotomous variable of "metro" and "non-metro," with metro as the reference category.

Statistical Analyses

We first ran Chi-square analyses to test the association between categorical predictors and both outcome variables. We intended to run hierarchical logistic regression models for both outcome variables. However, the bivariate analysis showed no statistically significant results for the question on how much preparation time Social Service Directors would need in order to provide one-on-one training to a social services colleague to "explain the social services' role in disaster planning and during a disaster", so we only ran a hierarchical logistic regression model for the "participate in disaster response planning and drills" question. The first step of the model included individual variables, and the second step added nursing home structural variables. We then ran an additional unanticipated regression model where we replaced the location variable of Coastal/non-Coastal with Wildfire/non-Wildfire. We conducted all analyses in IBM SPSS Version 26.

Results

Descriptive Statistics

A full description of the sample can be found in Bern-Klug et al. (2021). Broadly, the sample demographics are similar to national trends in nursing home social work: mostly female (93.1%, n = 523) and White (87.3%, n = 495). Slightly less than half were between the ages of 35–54 (45.9%, n = 258), one quarter were 18–34, (24.9%, n = 140), and the remainder were over the age of 55 (29.2%, n = 164). The majority of the sample was college educated: 47.8% (n = 267) reported a bachelor's degree as their highest level of education and 34.8% (n = 194) reported a master's degree. Just over half had a degree in social work either at the BSW or MSW level (55.6%, n = 310), but only a third had both a social work degree and a social work license (34.2%, n = 191), reflecting the lack of social work requirements for social service directors in nursing homes.

Social Service Involvement in Disaster Planning and Drills

Responses to the question, the extent to which social services staff "participate in disaster response planning and drills," indicated that the vast majority of social services departments participate in disaster training: 61.9% (n = 562) of respondents reported the department always participates, 20.3% (n = 184) usually, and 17.8% (n = 162) sometimes or never participated. In fact, only six percent reported that the social services department never participated in disaster response planning and drills.

Directors' Ability to Explain Social Services' Role in Disaster Planning and During a Disaster

The question about how much preparation time a social service director would need to explain the social services' role in disaster planning and during a disaster served as a proxy for whether the social service directors felt competent in their knowledge of disaster preparedness and response. Most directors felt fairly competent: 38.6% (n = 357) could explain the social services role with no preparation, 47% (n = 434) needed less than two hours to prepare. The remaining 11% either needed 10 or more hours to prepare (7%, n = 65) or felt that they could not do at all (4%, n = 37). We conducted bivariate analysis to determine whether structure or process variables influenced the social service director's preparedness. A lack of significant responses led us to conclude that they did not.

Table 1. Chi Square Test of Individual Predictors and Social Service Involvement in Disaster Preparedness and Response.

	X^2	df	p-value	N
Gender	2.36	2	.31	908
Race	2.48	2	.29	917
Education	5.48	4	.242	906
Experience	4.30	4	.37	915
Social Work License	1.30	2	.52	901

Chi-Square Models

Individual-Level Structures

Chi square tests were used for categorical predictors. Age of the social services director was a statistically significant predictor of always being involved in disaster planning and drills $X^2(4, N = 908) = 20.557, p < .001$, with the oldest nursing home social service directors most likely to be always involved. See Table 1 for the results of the other individual-level predictors, none of which showed evidence of statistical differences by group. [Insert Table 1 about here]

Nursing Home Structures

Among the nursing home level predictors, size of the nursing home predicted social services involvement in disaster planning and drills $X^2(4, N = 908) = 9.812, p = .04$ with social service workers in large size nursing homes (more than 120 beds) more likely to endorse that they were only never or sometimes involved.

Regression Model

Table 2 presents results from the hierarchical logistic regression model used to determine the likelihood that social workers were always involved in nursing home disaster preparedness and response, with individual-level and nursing home-level characteristics added at each step of the model. In step one, the individual-level characteristics were statistically significant, $X^2 (9) = 27.740$, $p = .002$. The model explained 4.0% (Nagelkerke $R2$) of the variance between being always involved (vs all other responses) in disaster preparedness and response and correctly classified 61.0% of cases. Age of the social service director was a statistically significant predictor of involvement in disaster preparedness and response. Compared to those age 55 and older, social service directors ages 18–34 (OR = .46, 95% CI [.29, .71], $p < .001$) and ages 35–54 (OR = .51, 95% CI [.36, .73], $p < .001$) were less likely to be involved in disaster preparedness and response. The addition of the nursing home level characteristics in the second step was not statistically significant. Step two added only

Table 2. Logistic Regression Model of Social Service Involvement in Disaster Preparedness and Response.

	Step One		Step 2	
	OR	95% CI	OR	95%CI
Gender (Male)	.84	[.50, 1.39]	.84	[.50, 1.41]
Age				
18–34	.46***	[.29, .71]	.45***	[.29, .70]
35–54	.51***	[.36, .73]	.50***	[.35, .73]
Race (White)	1.01	[.66, 1.55]	1.06	[.68, 1.66]
Education Level				
< 4 Year Degree	1.18	[.73, 1.90]	1.31	[.79, 2.20]
Bachelor Degree	.95	[.69, 1.31]	.99	[.71, 1.38]
Experience				
0–3 Years	.93	[.64, 1.37]	.93	[.62, 1.40]
4–9 Years	.81	[.56, 1.16]	.81	[.56, 1.17]
No Social Work License	.82	[.60, 1.12]	.81	[.59, 1.11]
Bed Size	–	–		
< 60 Beds			1.29	[.78, 2.15]
60–120 Beds			.95	[.67, 1.34]
Ownership	–	–	1.11	[.82, 1.51]
Rural/Urban	–	–	1.34	[.97, 1.88]
Staffing Ratio	–	–	.99	[.84, 1.17]
Region	–	–		
Northeast Coastal	–	–	1.15	[.72, 1.86]
South Coastal	–	–	1.10	[.76, 1.87]
Pacific Coastal	–	–	.92	[.52, 1.65]
Wildfire States †	–	–	.73	[.43, 1.23]

Note: UOR = Unadjusted Odds Ratio; AOR = Adjusted Odds Ratio; CI = Confidence Interval.
Reference Groups: Gender- Female; Age- 55+; Race- Other; Education Level- Master's Degree; Experience- more than 10 years; Bed Size- more than 120, Ownership- For profit, Rural/Urban- Urban, Staffing ration- continuous variable, Region- non-coastal; and Wildfire states- non-coastal.
† Census Regions were recoded into wildfire areas and included in a separate regression model in place of Coastal region.
*p < .05, **p < .01, ***p < .001

1.1% of additional explanation of the variance (Nagelkerke $R2$). No single nursing home characteristic was statistically significant in explaining variance. The unanticipated regression model with Coastal/non-Coastal replaced by Wildfire/non-Wildfire revealed no additional statistically significant findings. [Insert Table 2 about here]

Discussion

Our findings reveal that most nursing home social services departments (61.9%) are always involved in disaster planning and another 20.3% usually are – accounting for social services departments involvement in 80% of all U.S. Medicare and/or Medicaid certified nursing homes' disaster planning. Federal guidelines require nursing homes to train all of their staff every year on emergency and disaster plans (81 F.R. 68692, 2016), thus while not confirmed from this survey, it is likely the social services department is working with other departments in disaster planning. Interdisciplinary disaster planning would likely yield the best results for residents, because every department is impacted by a disaster, and all staff are needed for a comprehensive, multidimensional response. Interdisciplinary interventions in nursing homes have been shown to improve resident outcomes in other areas (Nazir et al., 2013). Strengthening federal guidelines for social service staffing and for interdisciplinary team participation in disaster planning is one structural change that might influence this process for nursing homes.

There are a number of limitations that should be considered when interpreting the findings of this study. First, methodologically, this data was collected using a self-report survey and reflects the perceptions of the social service directors who responded. Further, the outcome measure was double-barreled and may have inaccurately measured their participation. Future research should break out survey items. For example, "participate in disaster response planning" and "drills" could be listed as separate items to more accurately determine the nursing home social service departments' involvement in disaster planning. We also found that older social service directors were more likely to participate but we do not know their exact ages due to how the age was collected. We also do not know if age correlates to greater experience. Our only statistically significant result, age, was collected as a categorical variable. However, despite these limitations, this exploratory study of secondary data provides valuable insight into the involvement of social service directors and their staff in disaster preparedness of nursing homes.

Our statistical model was not successful in identifying structural predictors of social services departments' participation in disaster planning and drills. Indeed, neither characteristics of the social services director (other than the age of the director), nor the structural characteristics of the nursing home helped to explain the variation in social services department participation in disaster planning and drills. Our findings indicate that older nursing home social service directors were more likely to report their department was involved in disaster planning as compared with their younger counterparts. There is some research that found that social workers who remain in the profession are older (Wermeling, 2013) and that social workers who remain in the profession turnover frequently (Chiller & Crisp, 2012). Neither of these studies looked at nursing home social service directors. This would be interesting to explore further, to understand whether older social service directors have more experience, and as discovering the reasons might help nursing home administrators engage younger nursing home social service directors in disaster planning and drills. Understanding barriers to engagement among younger nursing home social service directors may also reveal training opportunities.

The data used in this study was collected pre-COVID. The COVID-19 global pandemic has been a completely different kind of disaster to which nursing homes have had to respond. During COVID-19 the roles of nursing home social service directors and their staffs have been similar to previous natural disasters such as facilitating communication between residents and their families and providing emotional support to both parties. In addition, the COVID-19 global pandemic has been prolonged, has left residents and staff particularly vulnerable to physical harm due to limited access to personal protective equipment (PPE), and has created additional psychosocial needs related to social isolation and separation from family members (e.g., Kusmaul et al., 2020). Since experts say that global pandemics may become more common in the future (David & Le Dévédec, 2019), disaster preparedness and response must incorporate the lessons learned from COVID-19, including the essential role of social service departments in disasters.

Implications for Social Work in Long Term Care

The most concerning part of our finding was that five percent of nursing home social service directors were never involved in disaster planning and drills and 12% were only sometimes involved. While these nursing homes are likely still engaged in disaster planning, the social service directors were absent from these activities. Due to all of the reasons discussed about how nursing home social service directors can contribute to a nursing home's disaster planning, this finding suggests that the absence of social workers from this process could be shaping the quality of the outcomes. While this study did not allow us to explore this possibility, this is a structural factor that is worth exploring in future research.

Previous studies on disaster preparedness in nursing homes have found that lack of personal knowledge about disasters and limited nursing home financial resources were cited as two of the most common barriers to preparedness and planning (Dosa et al., 2003). Social workers often feel unprepared to respond in the immediate aftermath of a disaster since few social workers are trained to act in a community-wide disaster (Newhill & Sites, 2000). While many social workers are not specifically trained in disaster preparedness, it is essential that social work education prepare all new social work professionals to be competent and ready to assist older adults during a disaster. This is particularly prevalent as so many social work roles intersect with older adults in disaster preparedness, response, and recovery.

The COVID-19 global pandemic and resultant impacts on nursing homes have shown us that social service workers are an important part of a nursing home's disaster response. COVID-19 has isolated residents from family members, and many residents have gotten sick and died. Social workers have been responsible for supporting isolated residents and concerned family members often with few resources because leadership and other disciplines have little understanding of what they do (Kusmaul et al., 2020; Miller et al., 2021). Moving forward, it will be important to understand the training and support needs of nursing home social workers, to ensure that they can fulfill their duty of supporting residents' well-being, resident rights, and dignity during disasters.

Additional research is needed on social workers in long-term care settings. Further research is necessary to explain why some nursing homes include their social services departments in disaster training and others do not. It is also important to document whether nursing homes that consistently include social services in disaster planning processes experience better disaster-related outcomes for residents. Future studies should investigate the role that nursing home social services staff members play in disaster planning and during a disaster.

Funding

Funding for data collection was provided by the RRF Foundation for Aging, in a grant to Mercedes Bern-Klug, University of Iowa.

ORCID

Nancy Kusmaul http://orcid.org/0000-0003-2278-8495
Allison Gibson http://orcid.org/0000-0002-4116-9465
Mercedes Bern-Klug http://orcid.org/0000-0001-6546-6141

References

Administration, 42 C.F.R. § 483.70 (2019). Office of the Federal Register (OFR) and the Government Publishing Office. https://www.ecfr.gov/cgi-bin/text-idx?SID=d224cefa707cdf deac2aa290bd4472d3&mc=true&node=sp42.5.483.b&rgn=div6#se42.5.483_140

Aldrich, N., & Benson, W. F. (2008). Disaster preparedness and the chronic disease needs of vulnerable older adults. *Preventing Chronic Disease*, 5(1), 1–7. https://www.cdc.gov/pcd/issues/2008/jan/pdf/07_0135.pdf

Bailey, G., Clark, E., Kaye, L., Torres, J., Nagle, P., Avery-Edwards, M., Frank, L., Hall, A. P., Kleinman, A., Miller, W., Morano, C., Dishler Shubin, S., Hines Smith, S., Whitaker, T., & Yagoda, L. (2003). *National Association of Social Workers Long-Term Care Facilities Standards Task Force*. National Association of Social Workers.

Behavioral Health Services, 42 C.F.R. § 483.40 (2016). Office of the Federal Register (OFR) and the Government Publishing Office. https://www.ecfr.gov/cgi-bin/text-idx?SID=d224cefa707cdfdeac2aa290bd4472d3&mc=true&node=sp42.5.483.b&rgn=div6#se42.5.483_140

Beltran, S., Luigi, P., & Kusmaul, N. (2020). Rising above the flood: Emergency management and gerontological social work. *Innovation in Aging*, 4(1), 65–66. https://doi.org/10.1093/geroni/igaa057.214

Bern-Klug, M., Smith, K., Roberts, A. R., Kusmaul, N., Gammonley, D., Hector, P., Hector, P., Hector, P., Bonifas, R., Herman, C., Downes, D., Munn, J., Rudderham, G., Cordes, E., & Connolly, R. (2021). About One-Third of Nursing Home Social Services Directors have Earned a Social Work Degree and License. *Journal of Gerontological Social Work*, 1–22. Advance Online Publication. https://doi.org/10.1080/01634372.2021.1891594

Bomba, P., Morrissey, M. B., & Leven, D. (2011). Key role of social work in effective communication and conflict resolution process: Medical Orders for Life-Sustaining Treatment
(MOLST) Program in New York and shared medical decision making at the end of life.
Journal of Social Work in End-of-Life & Palliative Care, 7(1), 56–82. https://doi.org/10.1080/
15524256.2011.548047

Brown, L., Rothman, M., & Norris, F. (2007). Issues in mental health care for older adults after
disasters. *Generations*, 31(4), 21–26.

Brown, L. M., Hyer, K., Schinka, J. A., Mando, A., Frazier, D., & Polivka-West, L. (2010). Use of
mental health services by nursing home residents after hurricanes. *Psychiatric Services*, 61
(1), 74–77. https://doi.org/10.1176/ps.2010.61.1.74

Castle, N. G., & Ferguson, J. C. (2010). What is nursing home quality and how is it measured?
The Gerontologist, 50(4), 426–442. https://doi.org/10.1093/geront/gnq052

Chiller, P., & Crisp, B. R. (2012). Sticking around: Why and how some social workers stay in
the profession. *Practice*, 24(4), 211–224.

Claver, M., Dobalian, A., Fickel, J., Ricci, K. A., & Horn Mallers, M. (2013). Comprehensive
care for vulnerable elderly veterans during disasters. *Archives of Gerontology and Geriatrics*,
56(1), 205–215. https://doi.org/10.1016/j.archger.2012.07.010

Council on Social Work Education. (2015). *Educational policy and accreditation standards for
baccalaureate and master's social work programs*. Author. https://cswe.org/getattachment/
Accreditation/Standards-and-Policies/2015-EPAS/2015EPASandGlossary.pdf.aspx

David, P.-M., & Le Dévédec, N. (2019). Preparedness for the next epidemic: Health and
political issues of an emerging paradigm. *Critical Public Health*, 29(3), 363–369. https://
doi.org/10.1080/09581596.2018.1447646

Donabedian, A. (1988). The quality of care: How can it be assessed? *JAMA*, 260(12),
1743–1748. https://doi.org/10.1001/jama.1988.03410120089033

Dosa, D., Feng, Z., Hyer, K., Brown, L. M., Thomas, K., & Mor, V. (2010). Effects of Hurricane
Katrina on nursing facility resident mortality, hospitalization, and functional decline.
Disaster Medicine and Public Health Preparedness, 4(1), S28. https://doi.org/10.1001/dmp.
2010.11

Dosa, D., Hyer, K., Thomas, K., Swaminathan, S., Feng, Z., Brown, L., & Mor, V. (2012). To
evacuate or shelter in place: Implications of universal hurricane evacuation policies on
nursing home residents. *Journal of the American Medical Directors Association*, 13(2),
190–e1. https://doi.org/10.1016/j.jamda.2011.07.011

Dosa, D. M., Samsonov, M. E., & Nace, D. A. (2003). A pilot study investigating bioterrorism
preparedness in area nursing homes. *JAGS*, 51(S4), S117. https://doi.org/10.1034/j.1600-
0889.2000.00001.x

Emergency Preparedness Requirements for Medicare and Medicaid Participating Providers
and Suppliers, 81 FR 63860 (September 16, 2016). Office of the Federal Register (OFR) and
the Government Publishing Office. https://www.govinfo.gov/content/pkg/FR-2016-09-16/
pdf/2016-21404.pdf

Fernandez, L.S., Byard, D., Lin, C-C., Benson, S., & Barbera, J.A. (2002). Frail elderly as disaster
victims: Emergency management strategies. *Prehospital and Disaster Medicine*, 17(2), 67–74.
https://doi.org/10.1017/S1049023X00000200

Frahm, K. A., Brown, L. M., & Gibson, M. (2012). The importance of end-of-life care in nursing
home settings is not diminished by a disaster. *OMEGA-Journal of Death and Dying*, 64(2),
143–155. https://doi.org/10.2190/OM.64.2.c

Goldman, E., & Galea, S. (2014). Mental health consequences of disasters. *Annual Review of
Public Health*, 35(1), 169–183. https://doi.org/https://doi.org/10.1146/annurev-publhealth
-032013-182435

Hamler, T. C., English, S. J., Beltran, S. J., & Miller, V. J. (2020). A Reflection of and Charge to Gerontological Social Work: Past Pandemics and the Current COVID-19 Crisis. *Journal of Gerontological Social Work*, *63*(6–7), 577–579. https://doi.org/10.1080/01634372.2020.1766629

Hepworth, D. H. Rooney, R. H., Rooney, G. D., Strom-Gottfried, K., & Larsen, J. (2013). Direct social work practice: Theory and skills (10th Ed). Belmont, CA: Brooks/Cole.

Holup, A. A., Hyer, K., Meng, H., & Volicer, L. (2017). Profile of nursing home residents admitted directly from home. *Journal of the American Medical Directors Association*, *18*(2), 131–137. https://doi.org/10.1016/j.jamda.2016.08.017

Hyer, K., Polivka-West, L., & Brown, L. (2007). Nursing homes and assisted living facilities: Planning and decision making for sheltering in place or evacuation. *Generations*, *31*(4), 29–33.

Kaiser Family Foundation (2019). *Average Number of Certified Nursing Facility Beds*. Author. Retrieved January 28, 2021 from https://www.kff.org/other/state-indicator/average-number-of-certified-nursing-facility-beds/?currentTimeframe=0&sortModel=%7B%22colId%22:%22Location%22,%22sort%22:%22asc%22%7D

Kusmaul, N., Bern-Klug, M., Heston-Mullins, J., Roberts, A. R., & Galambos, C. (2020). Nursing Home Social Work During COVID-19. *Journal of Gerontological Social Work*, *63*(6–7), 651–653. https://doi.org/10.1080/01634372.2020.1787577

Kusmaul, N., Gibson, A., & Leedahl, S. (2018). Gerontological Social Work Roles in Disaster Preparedness and Response. *Journal of Gerontological Social Work*, *61*(7), 692–696. https://doi.org/10.1080/01634372.2018.1510455

Ladika, S., Ladika, J., Xirasagar, S., Cornman, C., Davis, C., & Richter, J. (2008). Providing shelter to nursing home evacuees in disasters: Lessons from Hurricane Katrina. *American Journal of Public Health*, *98*(7), 1288–1293. https://doi.org/10.2105/AJPH.2006.107748

Lu, P., Kong, D., & Shelley, M. (2020). Making the Decision to Move to a Nursing Home: Longitudinal Evidence from the Health and Retirement Study. *Journal of Applied Gerontology*, 1–9. Office of the Federal Register (OFR) and the Government Publishing Office. https://doi.org/10.1177/0733464820949042

Miller, V. J., Hamler, T., Beltran, S., & Burns, J. (2021). Nursing home social services: A systematic review of the literature from 2010 to 2020. *Social Work in Health Care*, 1–23. [Advance Online Publication]. https://doi.org/https://doi.org/10.1080/00981389.2021.1908482

Naturale, A. (2007). Secondary traumatic stress in social workers responding to disasters: Reports from the field. *Clinical Social Work Journal*, *35*(3), 173–181. https://doi.org/10.1007/s10615-007-0089-1

Nazir, A., Unroe, K., Tegeler, M., Khan, B., Azar, J., & Boustani, M. (2013). Systematic review of interdisciplinary interventions in nursing homes. *Journal of the American Medical Directors Association*, *14*(7), 471–478. https://doi.org/10.1016/j.jamda.2013.02.005

Newhill, C., & Sites, E. (2000). Identifying human remains following an air disaster. *Social Work in Health Care*, *31*(4), 85–105. https://doi.org/10.1300/J010v31n04_06

Office of Inspector General (2006). *Nursing home emergency preparedness and response during recent hurricanes*. (OEI Publication No. 06- 06-00020).U.S. Department of Health and Human Services, Office of Inspector General. https://oig.hhs.gov/oei/reports/oei-06-06-00020.pdf

Office of Inspector General (2012a). *Gaps continue to exist in nursing home emergency preparedness and response during disasters: 2007-2010*. (OEI Publication No. 06- 09-00270).U.S. Department of Health and Human Services, Office of Inspector General. https://oig.hhs.gov/oei/reports/oei-06-09-00270.asp

Office of Inspector General (2012b). *Supplemental Information Regarding the Centers for Medicare & Medicaid Services' Emergency Preparedness Checklist for Health Care Facilities.* (OEI Publication No. 06- 09-00271).U.S. Department of Health and Human Services, Office of Inspector General.

Schnelle, J. F., Simmons, S. F., Harrington, C., Cadogan, M., Garcia, E., & Bates-Jensen, B., M. (2004). Relationship of nursing home staffing to quality of care. *Health Services Research, 39* (2), 225–250. https://doi.org/10.1111/j.1475-6773.2004.00225.x

Scoville, M. C. (1942). Wartime tasks of psychiatric social workers in Great Britain. *American Journal of Psychiatry, 99*(3), 358–363. https://doi.org/10.1176/ajp.99.3.358

Shippee, T., Hong, H., Henning-Smith, C., & Kane, R. (2015). Longitudinal changes in nursing home resident-reported quality of life: The role of facility characteristics. *Research on Aging, 37*(6), 555–580. https://doi.org/10.1177/0164027514545975

Simons, K. V. (2006). Organizational characteristics influencing nursing home social service directors' qualifications: A national study. *Health & Social Work, 31*(4), 266–274. https://doi.org/10.1093/hsw/31.4.266

Wermeling, L. (2013). Why social workers leave the profession: Understanding the profession and workforce. *Administration in Social Work, 37*(4), 329–339.

Social Service Directors' Roles and Self-Efficacy in Suicide Risk Management in US Nursing Homes

Xiaochuan Wang, Kelsey Simons, Denise Gammonley, Amy Restorick Roberts, and Mercedes Bern-Klug ⓘ

ABSTRACT

Nursing home (NH) residents have many risk factors for suicide in later life and transitions into and out of NHs are periods of increased suicide risk. The purpose of this study was to describe NH social service directors (SSDs) roles in managing suicide risk and to identify factors that influence self-efficacy in this area. This study used data from the 2019 National Nursing Home Social Services Directors survey (n = 924). One-fifth (19.7%) of SSDs reported a lack of self-efficacy in suicide risk management, as indicated by either needing significant preparation time or being unable to train others on intervening with residents at risk for suicide. Ordinal logistic regression identified SSDs who were master's prepared, reported insufficient social service staffing as a minor barrier (versus a major barrier) to psychosocial care, and those most involved in safety planning for suicide risk were more likely to report self-efficacy for training others. Implications include the need for targeted training of NH social service staff on suicide prevention, such as safety planning as an evidence-based practice. Likewise, sufficient staffing of qualified NH social service providers is critically important given the acute and chronic mental health needs of NH residents.

Suicide is the tenth leading cause of death in the US and suicide rates have steadily increased in the past decade (American Foundation for Suicide Prevention, 2019). Suicide rates are highest among middle-aged adults (45–64) and adults ages 75 and older, with men representing a disproportionate share of these deaths (Centers for Disease Control and Prevention & National Center for Injury Prevention and Control, 2019). As the baby boomer generation (adults born between 1946 and 1964) continues to reach the threshold of traditional retirement age (age 65) during the next decade, historically elevated suicide rates in this demographic are possible, if not likely (Conwell et al., 2011). Depression, functional impairment, illness, social isolation, loneliness, and access to lethal means (e.g., firearms) are among the most salient risk factors for suicide in adults 65 and over (Conwell et al., 2011; Van Orden & Conwell, 2011).

Healthcare providers are the front lines for late life suicide prevention. Older adults are more likely to be seen by healthcare professionals prior to suicide than younger adults (Ahmedani et al., 2014; Luoma et al., 2002); yet, studies suggest that suicide risk among older adults may go under-identified and under-treated (Arias et al., 2017; Simons et al., 2019). Stays in hospitals and in post-acute rehabilitation settings, such as nursing homes (NHs), are particularly important periods for identifying and addressing suicide risk in this age group (McCarthy et al., 2013; Mezuk et al., 2019; Szanto et al., 2013; Temkin-Greener et al., 2020). Such admissions, whether elective or emergent, may reflect changes in overall health that can be accompanied by decreased mood, poorer overall functioning, and adverse clinical outcomes (Dubljanin Raspopovic et al., 2014; Ghose et al., 2005; Watt et al., 2018). COVID-19 poses a particular challenge for NHs given use of visiting restrictions and social distancing measures that increase social isolation, which is a known risk factor for depression and suicide in older adults (Choi et al., 2015; National Academies of Sciences, Engineering, and Medicine 2020). Consequently, hospitalizations and post-acute stays in NHs are critical points for observations of patient mood, social functioning, and other risk factors for suicide, accompanied by interdisciplinary interventions to enhance psychosocial outcomes.

Approximately one-quarter (26.3%) of older adults who experience a Medicare-covered hospital stay are discharged to post-acute settings (e.g., NHs) rather than directly to the community (Werner & Konetzka, 2018). Despite being a 24-hour, supervised care environment, the incidence of death by suicide in NHs may be only marginally less common than suicide among community dwelling older adults (14.16 versus 15.66/100,000 per data from one US state) (Mezuk et al., 2015). Older adults in NHs experience more depression than their community-dwelling peers (Blazer, 2003). Transitions into and out of long-term care have been identified as risk periods for suicide, particularly for non-Hispanic white men (Mezuk et al., 2019). Within the Veterans Health Administration (VHA), suicide associated with NHs was found to be especially elevated within the first 3 weeks of discharge from this setting, when compared to an age and gender matched group of VHA patients who did not experience this type of care transition (McCarthy et al., 2013). Others have identified suicidal ideation among older adults in nursing homes as most common following admission and associated with clinical risk factors such as moderate to severe depression, aggressive behavior, psychiatric disorders, and pain that interferes with daily functions (Temkin-Greener et al., 2020). This prior research calls attention to the need to improve suicide risk management in the context of NH post-acute transitional care to ensure safety and well-being. However, there is relatively little knowledge regarding how suicide risk is managed in NHs and the competencies health care professionals possess for addressing acute mental health symptoms (e.g., severe depression, suicidal thoughts, and behaviors) among residents.

Nursing home social service roles and training in managing acute mental health symptoms

One-third of a national sample of 1,079 NHs reported inability to adequately meet nursing home residents' behavioral health service needs (Orth et al., 2019). Community NHs generally do not staff licensed, independent mental health professionals (e.g., psychologists, psychiatrists, and licensed clinical social workers) and most only contract with such providers for consultation as needed (Grabowski et al., 2010). However, NHs with 120 beds or more are required, per federal regulations, to staff social service providers to meet the overall psychosocial needs of residents (Bern-Klug et al., 2018). A majority of NHs, regardless of size, employ social service providers who meet federal regulatory requirements for qualifications (i.e., bachelor's in social work or similar degree in human services, plus 1 year of healthcare experience); (Roberts & Bowblis, 2017). Without direct access to licensed, independent mental health professionals, social workers and social service staff with training in mental health and aging may be among the most qualified to identify and address suicide risk among residents. The National Association of Social Work's (NASW) professional standards in long-term care facilities establish a key function of NH social service departments in ensuring, "health and mental health social work services are available to residents to assist with attaining or maintaining the highest practical mental and psychosocial well-being, while helping residents who display mental or psychosocial difficulty receive appropriate treatment and services" (National Association of Social Workers, 2003).

Depression and suicidal thoughts or behaviors, indicators of poor quality of life among older adults, are treatable conditions (Raue et al., 2017; Van Orden & Conwell, 2011) that NHs have a responsibility to identify and address. However, there is a lack of prior research regarding both NH social service staff's roles in managing mental health and suicide risk and research on roles of social workers in late life suicide prevention in general. There is also a wide range in educational credentials within the NH social service workforce, with some staff possessing less than bachelor's degrees (Bern-Klug et al., 2009), that could impact how well mental health issues are addressed in this setting. Prior research also suggests that increased staffing of social service providers in NHs reduces deficiencies in care related to quality of life (Bowblis & Roberts, 2020). The purpose of this study was twofold: 1) to describe NH social service director (SSD) roles in mental health care and in managing suicide risk and 2) to identify factors (professional characteristics, facility structural factors, and involvement in mental health and suicide risk management) that may influence SSDs' self-efficacy (i.e., perceived ability to instruct others) in suicide risk management.

Theoretical framework

This study is grounded in Bandura's theory of self-efficacy, the belief in one's ability to engage in particular behaviors in order to achieve a desired outcome. Self-efficacy provides a motivation to persevere in completing tasks and creates confidence about one's influence and success in achieving goals (Bandura, 1977, 1993). Self-efficacy develops in the context of relationships and contributes to perceived professional competence among health practitioners, such as perceived ability to resolve conflict in interprofessional teams (Sexton & Orchard, 2016). This study conceptualizes self-efficacy in managing suicide risk as SSDs' perceived ability to instruct other staff members in aspects of suicide risk assessment, intervention, and documentation. We propose that the perceived time needed for SSDs to prepare training reflects their self-confidence in the ability to train a fellow staff member in identifying and responding to suicide risk. Consistent with Bandura's theory, in this study we argue that the perceived time needed for SSDs to prepare training for suicide risk management may be a proxy for self-efficacy in one's own ability to intervene with residents at heightened risk for suicide. Social service staff educational attainment, training, and experience; clinical complexity among residents (e.g., % with SMI); and facility structural characteristics (e.g., ownership characteristics and barriers to psychosocial care) are all factors that have the potential to influence SSD departments' capacity to effectively address residents' psychosocial and mental health needs, thereby influencing SSDs' perceptions of self-efficacy to address suicide risk. This study was particularly focused on the impact of participation in mental health roles on self-efficacy for suicide risk management. Greater experience in mental health assessment (e.g., screening for depression) and the delivery of mental health interventions (e.g., safety planning and counseling or psychotherapy) are posited to create opportunities for applied skills that increase confidence (i.e., self-efficacy) for suicide risk management in accordance with Bandura's theory.

Materials and methods

This study draws on data from the 2019 National Nursing Home Social Services Director (NNHSSD) survey. Please see Bern-Klug et al. (2021) for a complete description of the methods. The survey asked a broad range of questions pertaining to topics such as SSDs' clinical and administrative roles in NHs, their training and educational backgrounds, perceived barriers to psychosocial care, interprofessional relationships, and characteristics of residents served. 924 SSDs completed the survey either online or by mail with an overall response rate of 30%. Facility characteristics (e.g., facility size, ownership type, and location) were extracted from the Centers for Medicare and Medicaid Services Provider of Services (CMS-POS) file and matched to participant data through unique participant IDs. The study was approved by the sponsoring university's institutional review board. Our study's focus on NH SSDs (versus all social service staff) reflects attention to the role of the director in providing leadership and oversight of processes and activities in suicide risk management. However, many NH social service departments are small and SSDs may be the only social service staff available or represent a sizable portion of such departments (Bern-Klug et al., 2021).

Measures

Social service directors' demographic and professional characteristics

Demographic data on gender (male, female, or non-binary), race (coded as White/Caucasian versus persons of color), Hispanic/Latino/Latinx ancestry (yes/no) and age (18–34, 35–54, or 55 and older) were obtained. In addition, SSDs were asked to indicate their highest level of education (less than a bachelor's, bachelor's, or master's degree), degree field (social work or other degree), social work licensure or certification status (yes/no), full-time employment status (35 hours per week as yes/no), and years of experience in NH social services (≤ 3 years, 4–9 years, or 10 or more years).

Facility characteristics including barriers to psychosocial care

Prior research has associated facility characteristics with quality outcomes and staffing in nursing homes (Bern-Klug et al., 2021; Comondore et al., 2009; Harrington et al., 2012; Konetzka et al., 2015). These factors could potentially impact on SSDs' perceived ability to address the residents' psychosocial and mental health needs and to intervene with residents at greater suicide risk. To control for these factors, the following facility information was extracted from the CMS-POS file: number of beds (< 60, 60–120, 121 or more), participation in Medicare or Medicaid (both Medicare and Medicaid, or only one), ownership status (for-profit versus other status), part of a chain of two or more nursing homes (yes/no), location (metropolitan versus non-metropolitan area), and Census region (Northeast, Midwest, South, or West). In addition, information on whether the facility contracts with a provider for mental health services (yes/no, or don't know) was obtained through the survey. Participating SSDs were also asked to provide an estimate of the total percentage of residents with a serious mental illness (SMI) within their NHs, such as schizophrenia, bipolar disorder, severe depression or severe post-traumatic stress disorder (PTSD) (< 10%, 10–24%, 25–49%, 50% or more, or don't know). Responses coded as don't know were treated as missing in our study. Two items addressed facility-related barriers to SSDs' ability to adequately attend to residents' psychosocial and mental health needs: 1) Insufficient professional supervision or consultation to guide/support social services and 2) Not enough social service staff for the number of residents. These items are rated on a 4-point scale (1 = not a barrier, 2 = minor barrier, 3 = moderate barrier, 4 = major barrier).

Roles in mental health and suicide risk management

Participants were also asked the extent to which social services was involved in each of the following six activities: 1) screens for anxiety; 2) screens for depression; 3) creates a safety plan for residents at risk of suicide; 4) provides counseling (psychotherapy) directly to residents with depression and/or mood disorder; 5) refers residents to a mental health professional for individual counseling; and 6) decides when to transfer a resident to a psychiatric unit (1 = social services is never involved, 2 = social services is sometimes involved, 3 = social services is usually involved, 4 = social services is always involved, or 5 = not done at our facility). For our analyses, responses were recoded as usually/always involved versus never/sometimes involved or not done at the facility. Participants were also asked to indicate: 7) whether they were responsible for completing the Patient Health Questionnaire (PHQ) depression screen (yes/no) contained within the mandated Minimum Data Set (MDS) resident assessment instrument (Saliba et al., 2012).

Dependent variable – self-efficacy for suicide risk management

SSDs' self-efficacy for suicide risk management was indicated by the following single-item question: "Please estimate how much preparation time you would need to provide one-on-one training to a social services colleague about how to assess suicide risk in residents who are depressed, develop (and carry out) a safety plan, and provide appropriate documentation in the chart." Response options included: 1 = could do without prep time, 2 = would need up to 2 hours of prep time, 3 = would need up to 10 hours of prep time, and 4 = not able to do. Responses were reverse coded so higher values indicate greater self-efficacy in suicide risk management. For the purpose of this study, participants indicating they needed significant prep time were combined with those stating they were not able to engage in this activity.

Data analysis

Descriptive analyses were conducted to provide a summary of the sample characteristics. Bivariate associations between each independent variable and SSDs' self-efficacy in suicide risk management were examined using chi-square tests. An ordinal logistic regression was performed to examine the association (odds ratios [ORs], 95% confidence intervals [CIs], and significance levels) between SSDs' demographic and professional characteristics, facility characteristics, care barriers, social service roles, and self-reported competency in suicide risk management. Multicollinearity of independent variables was examined using variance inflation factor (VIF) and was not found to be an issue. The proportional odds assumption was examined using Test of Parallel Lines in SPSS, and was satisfied with a non-significant chi-square statistic result ($\chi^2(40) = 30.91$; $p = .85$). All statistical analyses were conducted using SPSS Version 25.

Results

Sample and facility characteristics

Table 1 presents descriptive results of NH SSDs' demographic and professional characteristics and facility structural factors. Approximately half of the participants were ages 35–54 years old (47.4%), possessed 10 years of experience in NH social services (47.1%), and were bachelor's-level practitioners (49.0%). A majority had social work degrees (57.9%). About half (47.4%) reported holding a state license/certification in social work, including some respondents who lacked a social work degree. Most were employed by NHs that were for-profit (62.7%), part of a chain (2 or more owned or leased facilities) (58.1%) and received Medicare and Medicaid reimbursement (95.2%). 41.2% of SSDs were employed in NHs located in the Midwest census region, followed by 29.1% from the South region, 16.0% from the Northeast, and 13.7% from the West. 40.2% of SSDs reported fewer than 10% of residents in their NHs possessed SMI; whereas 30.8% reported 25% or more of their residents possessed such disorders. Most NHs had contracts with an outside agency or individuals to provide mental health and/or behavioral health services to residents (88.8%) and relatively few of these services were provided off-site (17.9%).

Bivariate associations between study variables and self-efficacy for suicide risk management

Table 2 presents the characteristics of SSDs and the NHs in which they were employed, stratified by SSDs' self-reported competency for suicide risk management. Nearly one-third of SSDs (30.9%) reported they would be able to provide one-on-one training to a social services colleague on suicide risk management without any preparation time. Approximately one-half (49.4%) believed they would be able to conduct the training but would need some preparation time (up to 2 hours). The remaining SSDs (19.7%) perceived themselves being less confident to provide training about suicide risk management, as indicated by either needing significant preparation time or being unable to do this at all. SSDs' self-reported competency for suicide risk

Table 1. Descriptive statistics of study variables.

Variable	N	%	Valid N
Demographics and professional characteristics			
Gender			917
Male	69	7.5	
Female	845	92.1	
Non-binary	3	0.3	
Race			910
White/Caucasian	802	88.1	
Persons of Color	108	11.9	
Hispanic/Latino/Latinx origin (No)	872	95.5	913
Age			914
18-34	257	28.1	
35-54	433	47.4	
55 and up	224	24.5	
Years of experience in NHSS			921
<1-3 years	243	26.4	
4-9 years	244	26.5	
10+ years	434	47.1	
Educational attainment			912
<4 year degree	142	15.6	
Bachelor's degree	447	49.0	
Master's degree	323	35.4	
Social Work degree (Yes)	528	57.9	912
Social Work license/certification (Yes)	429	47.4	906
Fulltime employment (35+ hours/week, Yes)	858	93.3	920
Facility characteristics			
Ownership status (For profit, Yes)	572	62.7	913
Program Participation			913
Medicare and Medicaid	869	95.2	
Medicare only or Medicaid only	44	4.8	
In metropolitan area (Yes)	611	66.1	913
Contracts with MH provider (Yes)	810	88.8	912
Chain status (Yes)	530	58.1	913
Bed size			913
<60 beds	182	19.9	
60-120	483	52.9	
121 or more	248	27.2	
Percentage of residents with SMI			915
Census Region			
Northeast	146	16.0	913
Midwest	376	41.2	
South	266	29.1	
West	125	13.7	
MH services provided off-site to residents (Yes)	163	17.9	913

Note. NH= nursing home; SS= social services; MH= mental health; SMI= serious mental illness.

management significantly differed by SSDs' age ($\chi^2(4) = 10.97$; $p = .027$), educational attainment ($\chi^2(4) = 31.85$; $p < .001$), possession of social work degree ($\chi^2(2) = 6.04$; $p = .049$), whether the facility was located in metropolitan area ($\chi^2(2) = 7.79$; $p = .02$), and the number of beds in the facility ($\chi^2(4) = 10.56$; $p = .032$).

Table 3 presents the distribution of SSDs' perceived facility barriers to psychosocial care and social services role involvement by self-efficacy in suicide risk management. SSDs' self-efficacy in suicide risk management

Table 2. Sample characteristics by self-reported competency for suicide risk management.

Variable	Need significant prep or not able to do n = 177 (19.7%)	Could do with some prep n = 443 (49.4%)	Could do without prep n = 277 (30.9%)	χ2 (df)	p
Demographics and professional characteristics					
Gender				0.81(2)	.67
Female	161 (91.5)	405 (91.8)	257 (93.5)		
Male/ Non-binary	15 (8.5)	36 (8.2)	18 (6.5)		
Race				1.32(2)	.52
White/Caucasian	155 (88.6)	380 (87.0)	246 (89.8)		
Persons of Color	20 (11.4)	57 (13.0)	28 (10.2)		
Hispanic/Latino/Latinx origin (No)	168 (95.5)	418 (95.2)	264 (96.4)	0.53(2)	.77
Age				10.97(4)	.027
18–34	43 (24.4)	128 (29.1)	76 (27.7)		
35–54	74 (42.0)	212 (48.2)	141 (51.5)		
55 and up	59 (33.5)	100 (22.7)	57 (20.8)		
Years of experience in NHSS				1.61(4)	.81
<1-3 years	48 (27.1)	122 (27.5)	65 (23.6)		
4–9 years	47 (26.6)	114 (25.7)	78 (28.3)		
10+ years	82 (46.3)	207 (46.7)	133 (48.2)		
Educational attainment				31.85(4)	<.001
<4 year degree	41 (23.6)	65 (14.8)	32 (11.7)		
Bachelor's degree	84 (48.3)	239 (54.4)	113 (41.2)		
Master's degree	49 (28.2)	135 (30.8)	129 (47.1)		
Social Work degree (Yes)	89 (51.1)	250 (56.9)	172 (62.8)	6.04(2)	.049
Social Work license/certification (Yes)	78 (45.1)	204 (46.8)	135 (49.5)	0.89(2)	.64
Fulltime employment (35+ hours/week, Yes)	163 (92.1)	410 (92.6)	262 (94.9)	1.94(2)	.38
Facility characteristics					
Ownership status (For profit, Yes)	102 (58.0)	272 (62.2)	181 (66.3)	3.24(2)	.20
Program Participation				1.59(2)	.45
Medicare or Medicaid only	11 (6.3)	21 (4.8)	10 (3.7)		
Medicare and Medicaid	165 (93.8)	416 (95.2)	263 (96.3)		
In metropolitan area (Yes)	106 (60.2)	286 (65.4)	198 (72.5)	7.79(2)	.02
Contracts with MH provider (Yes)	148 (84.6)	391 (88.7)	251 (91.6)	5.31(2)	.07

(*Continued*)

Table 2. (Continued).

| Variable | Self-reported competency for suicide risk management, No. (%) | | | | | |
	Need significant prep or not able to do n = 177 (19.7%)	Could do with some prep n = 443 (49.4%)	Could do without prep n = 277 (30.9%)	χ2 (df)	p
Chain status (Yes)	101 (57.4)	250 (57.2)	163 (59.7)	0.47(2)	.79
Bed size					
<60 beds	43 (24.4)	88 (20.1)	45 (16.5)	10.56(4)	.032
60–120	99 (56.3)	232 (53.1)	140 (51.3)		
121 or more	34 (19.3)	117 (26.8)	88 (32.2)		
Percentage of residents with SMI				2.92(6)	.82
<10%	74 (42.3)	179 (40.7)	104 (38.0)		
10%–24%	48 (27.4)	132 (30.0)	77 (28.1)		
25%–49%	29 (16.6)	73 (16.6)	57 (20.8)		
50% or more	24 (13.7)	56 (12.7)	36 (13.1)		
Census Region				1.43(6)	.96
Northeast	25 (14.2)	72 (16.5)	45 (16.5)		
Midwest	75 (42.6)	183 (41.9)	107 (39.2)		
South	50 (28.4)	124 (28.4)	84 (30.8)		
West	26 (14.8)	58 (13.3)	37 (13.6)		
MH services provided off-site to residents (Yes)	33 (18.8)	80 (18.3)	47 (17.2)	0.21(2)	.90

Note. NH = nursing home; SS = social services; MH = mental health; SMI = serious mental illness.

Table 3. Summary of facility barriers and social services roles by self-reported competency for suicide risk management.

Variable	Self-reported competency for suicide risk management, No. (%)			$\chi2$ (df)	p
	Need significant prep or not able to do n = 177 (19.7%)	Could do with some prep n = 443 (49.4%)	Could do without prep n = 277 (30.9%)		
Facility barriers to psychosocial care					
Insufficient consultation/ supervision				13.88(6)	.031
Not a barrier	62 (35.0)	181 (41.3)	134 (48.7)		
Minor barrier	54 (30.5)	126 (28.8)	74 (26.9)		
Moderate barrier	37 (20.9)	93 (21.2)	38 (13.8)		
Major barrier	24 (13.6)	38 (8.7)	29 (10.5)		
Not enough SS staff for the number of residents				8.08(6)	.23
Not a barrier	68 (38.4)	156 (35.4)	100 (36.4)		
Minor barrier	30 (16.9)	118 (26.8)	66 (24.0)		
Moderate barrier	33 (18.6)	81 (18.4)	53 (19.3)		
Major barrier	46 (26.0)	86 (19.5)	56 (20.4)		
Social services roles					
Screen for anxiety				16.94(2)	<.001
Usually/always involved	111 (62.7)	345 (78.4)	211 (76.2)		
Other (never/sometimes involved or not done)	66 (37.3)	95 (21.6)	66 (23.8)		
Screen for depression				21.68(2)	<.001
Usually/always involved	140 (79.1)	397 (90.0)	257 (92.8)		
Other (never/sometimes involved or not done)	37 (20.9)	44 (10.0)	20 (7.2)		
Create safety plan for residents at risk of suicide				26.49(2)	<.001
Usually/always involved	119 (67.2)	366 (83.2)	236 (85.5)		
Other (never/sometimes involved or not done)	58 (32.8)	74 (16.8)	40 (14.5)		
Provide counseling (psychotherapy) directly				2.19(2)	.33
Usually/always involved	83 (46.9)	231 (52.6)	148 (53.6)		
Other (never/sometimes involved or not done)	94 (53.1)	208 (47.4)	128 (46.4)		
Refer residents to mental health professionals				7.50(2)	.023
Usually/always involved	158 (89.3)	415 (93.9)	265 (95.7)		
Other (never/sometimes involved or not done)	19 (10.7)	27 (6.1)	12 (4.3)		
Help decide on psychiatric hospitalization				15.03(2)	.001
Usually/always involved	138 (78.0)	389 (88.2)	249 (89.9)		
Other (never/sometimes involved or not done)	39 (22.0)	52 (11.8)	28 (10.1)		
Section D (Mood) of MDS completed by SS (Yes)	162 (91.5)	423 (95.5)	270 (97.5)	8.61(2)	.013

Note. SS = social services; MDS = Minimum Data set.

varied significantly by the extent to which they considered insufficient consultation or supervision as one facility barrier to providing psychosocial care ($\chi^2(6) = 13.88$; $p = .031$). Additionally, SSDs' self-reported competency for suicide risk management differed significantly depending on the degree of social services role involvement in six activities, including anxiety screening

Table 4. Results of ordinal logistic regression on self-reported competency for suicide risk management (N = 811).

Variables		OR (95% CI)
Gender (Ref = Female)	Male/ Non-binary	0.83 (0.50, 1.37)
Race (Ref = White/Caucasian)	Persons of color	0.72 (0.46, 1.11)
Hispanic/Latino/Latinx origin (Ref = No)	Yes	0.77 (0.38, 1.55)
Age (Ref = 18–34 years old)	55 years and older	0.73 (0.48, 1.12)
	35–54 years old	1.18 (0.82, 1.69)
Years of experience in NHSS	10+ years	1.05 (0.71, 1.56)
(Ref = <1-3 years)	4–9 years	1.12 (0.76, 1.64)
Educational attainment	<4 year degree	0.56 (0.33, 0.97)*
(Ref = Master's degree)	Bachelor's degree	0.57 (0.41, 0.79)**
Social Work degree (Ref = Yes)	No	0.90 (0.64, 1.27)
Social Work license/certification (Ref = No)	Yes	0.93 (0.68, 1.28)
Full time employment (Ref = Yes)	No	1.16 (0.64, 2.12)
Ownership type (Ref = For profit)	Government/nonprofit	0.81 (0.59, 1.11)
Program participation (Ref = Medicare and Medicaid)	Only one program	0.68 (0.35, 1.33)
In metropolitan area (Ref = Yes)	No	0.85 (0.62, 1.17)
Contracts with MH provider (Ref = Yes)	No	0.77 (0.49, 1.19)
Chain status (Ref = Yes)	No	1.01 (0.75, 1.35)
Bed size (Ref = less than 60 beds)	121 or more	1.35 (0.83, 2.19)
	60–120	0.99 (0.66, 1.47)
Percentage of residents with SMI	10%-24%	1.07 (0.77, 1.50)
(Ref = less than 10%)	25–49%	1.27 (0.85, 1.89)
	50% or more	1.21 (0.77, 1.90)
MH services provided off-site (Ref = Yes)	No	0.97 (0.68, 1.38)
Region (Ref = Midwest)	Northeast	0.77 (0.49, 1.19)
	South	0.94 (0.66, 1.33)
	West	0.90 (0.57, 1.43)
Insufficient consultation/supervision	Not a barrier	1.10 (0.65, 1.86)
(Ref = Major barrier)	Minor barrier	0.85 (0.51, 1.44)
	Moderate barrier	0.75 (0.43, 1.28)
Not enough SS staff for the number of residents	Not a barrier	1.33 (0.88, 2.02)
(Ref = Major barrier)	Minor barrier	1.63 (1.07, 2.47)*
	Moderate barrier	1.37 (0.88, 2.14)
Screen for anxiety (Ref = Usually/always involved)	Other	1.19 (0.80, 1.76)
Screen for depression (Ref = Usually/always involved)	Other	0.63 (0.35, 1.10)
Create safety plan (Ref = Usually/always involved)	Other	0.66 (0.44, 0.97)*
Provide counseling sessions	Other	0.92 (0.69, 1.23)
(Ref = Usually/always involved)		
Refer to MH professionals	Other	0.69 (0.37, 1.30)
(Ref = Usually/always involved)		
Decide on psychiatric hospitalization	Other	0.68 (0.44, 1.05)
(Ref = Usually/always involved)		
Section D (Mood) of MDS completed by SS	No	0.76 (0.37, 1.57)
(Ref = Yes)		
Salary		1.06 (0.96, 1.17)

Note. NH = nursing home; SS = social services; MH = mental health; SMI = serious mental illness; MDS = Minimum Data set. $*p < .05$; $**p < .01$; $***p < .001$

($\chi^2(2) = 16.94$; $p < .001$), depression screening ($\chi^2(2) = 21.68$; $p < .001$), creation of safety plans for residents who were at risk of suicide ($\chi^2(2) = 26.49$; $p < .001$), referral of residents to mental health professionals for individual counseling ($\chi^2(2) = 7.50$; $p = .023$), help with decision on psychiatric hospitalization ($\chi^2(2) = 15.03$; $p = .001$), and completion of Section D (Mood) of MDS ($\chi^2(2) = 8.61$; $p = .013$).

Factors associated with self-efficacy for suicide risk management

An ordinal regression model was utilized to examine the association between each independent variable and SSDs' self-efficacy for suicide risk management. Model significance was examined. A significant improvement in the fit of final model over the null model was observed ($\chi^2(40)$ = 93.45; $p < .001$). Three variables emerged as statistically significant factors. As shown in Table 4, SSDs whose highest educational attainment was less than a bachelor's degree (OR = 0.56, 95% CI [0.33, 0.97], $p = .037$) or a bachelor's degree (OR = 0.57, 95% CI [0.41, 0.79], $p = .001$) were less likely to report greater self-efficacy (i.e., could do with no or some preparation time versus need significant preparation time or not able to do) to provide one-on-one training to a social services colleague about suicide risk management when compared to their counterparts who held a master's degree. Respondents who perceived having insufficient social service staff as a minor barrier were more likely to perceive self-efficacy in suicide risk management than those who considered it as major barrier (OR = 1.63, 95% CI [1.07, 2.47], $p = .022$), controlling for all other variables. Compared with those who reported that social services was usually or always involved in safety planning for residents at risk of suicide, respondents who indicated that this activity was not done in their facilities or social services was never or only sometimes involved in this activity were less likely to perceive greater competence in suicide risk management (OR = 0.66, 95% CI [0.44, 0.97], $p = .036$).

Discussion

This study aimed to describe nursing home SSDs role involvement in activities related to managing suicide risk and identify factors associated with self-efficacy in suicide risk management. This study identified SSDs as typically engaged in screening residents for mental health conditions (e.g., anxiety and depression), creating safety plans for residents at risk for suicide, and providing coordination of care for those with identified mental health needs (e.g., referrals to mental health providers or transfers to inpatient care). Likewise, while many reported a sense of confidence to train others in managing suicide risk (i.e., some or no preparation time required), approximately one-fifth of the SSDs reported either needing significant preparation time to provide such one-to-one training or a lack of confidence to engage in this activity. Three factors emerged as positively associated with this perception of self-efficacy in suicide risk management in multivariate analysis: possessing an advanced degree (master's vs. bachelor's/less than bachelor's prepared); insufficient social service staffing as only a minor barrier to psychosocial care; and SSD involvement in safety planning for suicide risk.

Our findings are consistent with prior studies of gerontological social workers and nurses, including those employed by nursing homes. For example, NH social workers reflecting upon their role and experiences, have identified the work environment as challenging, requiring a broad range of coping skills, mattering to the facility and to the lives of residents, and resulting in a sense of accomplishment (Ahyoung et al., 2016). Gerontological social workers who have opportunities to work with clients with complex or chronic care needs, to help their clients navigate systems, and to influence such service systems, report stronger professional self-efficacy (Bonifas et al., 2012). Intention to deliver psychosocial interventions to NH residents with problematic dementia behaviors is positively influenced by stronger perceived self-efficacy among nurses (Ludwin & Meeks, 2018). Nurse self-efficacy has been identified as more important than acquiring knowledge in promoting the implementation of advance care planning activities (Gilissen et al., 2020).

Provider self-efficacy has also been associated with perceived effectiveness to respond to suicidal behaviors among providers in non-NH settings. Betz et al. (2013) noted higher self-confidence in suicide screening skills but less confidence in assessing risk severity and providing counseling among emergency department nurses and physicians. In one study, behavioral health clinicians who reported greater self-efficacy to assess and respond to suicide risk demonstrated improved clinical practice skills for responding to suicidal behavior as presented in training vignettes (Lee et al., 2016). Behavioral health clinicians with a higher level of self-efficacy in relation to assessing suicide risk have also reported less anxiety and discomfort about working with suicidal persons (Mitchell et al., 2020).

Implications for training and staffing

Our study identified a potential need for further training and skills development among NH SSDs in suicide risk management, particularly among those who lack advanced degrees. In relation to roles in mental health services, being usually or always involved in creating safety plans enhanced feelings of self-efficacy for training other staff in how to identify and address suicide risk within their facilities. Safety planning is a standardized, cognitive-behavioral intervention and best practice for suicide prevention (Stanley et al., 2018). It can also be adapted for working with older adults, including those in NHs (Conti et al., 2020).

As a result of this finding, social work training programs and organizations (e.g., National Association of Social Workers) should consider offering workshops to train NH social service professionals in the development and implementation of safety planning for their residents. This may be particularly important during the era of COVID-19, when visiting restrictions have contributed to growing social isolation of NH residents. Social isolation is a significant contributor to both suicide (Conwell et al., 2011; Van Orden & Conwell, 2011) and all-cause mortality in older adults (National Academies of

Sciences, Engineering, and Medicine 2020). It was also posited to have contributed to increased suicides among older adults in Hong Kong during the Severe Acute Respiratory Syndrome (SARS) epidemic of 2003 (Cheung et al., 2008). Van Orden et al. (2020) have adapted a similar cognitive-behavioral approach as safety planning to address a need for social connection planning among older adults during COVID-19.

A second finding relates to the need for sufficient staffing of qualified NH social service personnel in order to manage the acute and chronic mental health needs of residents. In this study, nearly one-third of respondents reported 25% or more of their NH's residents had an SMI diagnosis. National estimates indicate the prevalence of SMI (those with bipolar disorder, schizophrenia, and psychotic disorder) in NHs is 20% (Preadmission Screening and Resident Review (PASRR) Technical Assistance Center, 2019). A recent national study identified social service staffing is actually lower in facilities with a high population of residents with SMI compared to facilities that have fewer residents with SMI (Jester et al., 2020). Appropriate mental health and social services are necessary to meet the high psychosocial care needs of residents with SMI, as they are often younger and more likely to become long-stay residents if admitted (Aschbrenner et al., 2011; Grabowski et al., 2009). Likewise, dementia is highly common in this setting – present in up to 58% of NH residents nationally, and the majority of these residents are affected by the behavioral and psychological symptoms of dementia (Grabowski et al., 2009; Seitz et al., 2010). Social service staff with higher qualifications are able to improve care through reducing residents' behavioral symptoms and avoiding the use of antipsychotic medications (Roberts et al., 2020).

In this study, approximately 40% of SSDs reported insufficient social service staffing as a moderate or major barrier in relation to the number of residents. When comparing staffing levels across different NH departments, social services is quite low (Harris-Kojetin et al., 2019) and has experienced the smallest increases in staffing levels over time (Roberts et al., 2019). Nevertheless, research has shown that higher qualifications and higher staffing levels of social service staff improve NH quality (Vongxaiburana et al., 2011). In addition, increasing the staffing level of social services is an efficient and cost-effective approach to improve quality of care and quality of life (Bowblis & Roberts, 2020a). Similarly, those who reported social service staffing as only a minor barrier to providing psychosocial services in their NHs were more likely to report confidence in training others to identify and address suicide risk among residents. Clearly, there is a serious need for adequate staffing, along with SSDs who are empowered to provide leadership and services to proactively address suicide risk management.

Limitations and strengths

A limitation of this study is its use of single-item indicators of constructs of interest, including our main outcome of self-efficacy for suicide risk management. Likewise, self-perception of the amount of time necessary to train a colleague is a subjective rating of this outcome that does not address actual competency for performing the task. As a cross-sectional study, statistically significant associations between predictors and the outcome of interest cannot be interpreted as causality. Other factors not measured, such as SSDs receiving training in this area previously, involvement in professional networks, or personal biases and views about death and dying could influence feelings of competence regarding suicide risk management. Despite these limitations, this was the first known study pertaining to NH SSDs self-efficacy for engaging in suicide prevention. As social service staff fulfill critical roles as providers of psychosocial services in NHs, knowledge of their roles in mental health is important information for quality improvement and continuing education, particularly during this era of COVID-19 when infection control strategies have socially isolated NH residents.

Acknowledgments

The authors would like to acknowledge the statistical support provided by Kevin M. Smith, University of Iowa, Department of Psychological and Quantitative Foundations.

ORCID

Mercedes Bern-Klug ⓘ http://orcid.org/0000-0001-6546-6141

Declaration of interest statement

The authors have no conflicts of interests to report

References

Ahmedani, B. K., Simon, G. E., Stewart, C., Beck, A., Waitzfelder, B. E., Rossom, R., Lynch, F., Owen-Smith, A., Hunkeler, E. M., Whiteside, U., Operskalski, B. H., Coffey, M. J., & Solberg, L. I. (2014). Health care contacts in the year before suicide death. *Journal of General Internal Medicine*, *29*(6), 870–877. https://doi.org/10.1007/s11606-014-2767-3

Ahyoung, A. L., Lee, S. N., & Armour, M. (2016). Drivers of change: Learning from the lived experiences of nursing home social workers. *Social Work in Health Care*, *55*(3), 247–264. https://doi.org/10.1080/00981389.2015.1111967

American Foundation for Suicide Prevention. (2019). *Suicide Statistics*. Retrieved https://afsp.org/suicide-statistics

Arias, S. A., Boudreaux, E. D., Segal, D. L., Miller, I., Camargo, C. A., Jr., & Betz, M. E. (2017). Disparities in treatment of older adults with suicide risk in the emergency department. *Journal of the American Geriatrics Society*, 65(10), 2272–2277. https://doi.org/10.1111/jgs. 15011

Aschbrenner, K., Grabowski, D. C., Cai, S., Bartels, S. J., & Mor, V. (2011). Nursing home admissions and long-stay conversions among persons with and without serious mental illness. *Journal of Aging & Social Policy*, 23(3), 286–304. https://doi.org/10.1080/08959420. 2011.579511

Bandura, A. (1977). Self-efficacy: Toward a unifying theory of behavioral change. *Psychological Review*, 84(2), 191–215. https://doi.org/10.1037//0033-295x.84.2.191

Bandura, A. (1993). Perceived self-efficacy in cognitive development and functioning. *Educational Psychologist*, 28(2), 117–148. https://doi.org/10.1207/s15326985ep2802_

Bern-Klug, M., Byram, E., Sabbagh Steinberg, N., Gamez Garcia, H., & Burke, K. C. (2018). Nursing home residents' legal access to onsite professional psychosocial care: Federal and state regulations do not meet minimum professional social work standards. *The Gerontologist*, 58(4), e260–e272. https://doi.org/10.1093/geront/gny053

Bern-Klug, M., Kramer, K. W., Chan, G., Kane, R., Dorfman, L. T., & Saunders, J. B. (2009). Characteristics of nursing home social services directors: How common is a degree in social work? *Journal of the American Medical Directors Association*, 10(1), 36–44. https://doi.org/ 10.1016/j.jamda.2008.06.011

Bern-Klug, M., Smith, K. M., Roberts, A. R., Kusmaul, N., Gammonley, D., Hector, P., Simons, K., Galambos, C., Bonifas, R., Herman, C., Downes, D., Munn, J. C., Rudderham, G., Cordes, E. A., & Connolly, R. (2021). About a third of nursing home social services directors have earned a social work degree and license. *Journal of Gerontological Social Work*, 1–22. https://doi.org/10.1080/01634372.2021.1891594

Betz, M. E., Sullivan, A. F., Manton, A. P., Espinola, J. A., Miller, I., Camargo, C. A., Jr., . . . Investigators, E.-S. (2013). Knowledge, attitudes, and practices of emergency department providers in the care of suicidal patients. *Depression and Anxiety*, 30(10), 1005–1012. https:// doi.org/10.1002/da.22071

Blazer, D. G. (2003). Depression in late life: Review and commentary. *The Journals of Gerontology. Series A, Biological Sciences and Medical Sciences*, 58(3), 249–265. https://doi. org/10.1093/gerona/58.3.m249

Bonifas, R., Gammonley, D., & Simons, K. (2012). Gerontological social workers' perceived efficacy for influencing client outcomes. *Journal of Gerontological Social Work*, 55(6), 519–536. https://doi.org/10.1080/01634372.2012.690837

Bowblis, J. R., & Roberts, A. R. (2020). Cost-effective adjustments to nursing home staffing to improve quality. *Medical Care Research and Review*, 77(3), 274–284. https://doi.org/10.1177/ 1077558718778081

Centers for Disease Control and Prevention, & National Center for Injury Prevention and Control. (2019). *Web-based injury statistics query and reporting system (WISQARS)*. Retrieved https://www.cdc.gov/injury/wisqars/index.html

Cheung, Y. T., Chau, P. H., & Yip, P. S. (2008). A revisit on older adults suicides and Severe Acute Respiratory Syndrome (SARS) epidemic in Hong Kong. *International Journal of Geriatric Psychiatry*, 23(12), 1231–1238. https://doi.org/10.1002/gps.2056

Choi, H., Irwin, M. R., & Cho, H. J. (2015). Impact of social isolation on behavioral health in elderly: Systematic review. *World Journal of Psychiatry*, 5(4), 432–438. https://doi.org/10. 5498/wjp.v5.i4.432

Comondore, V. R., Devereaux, P. J., Zhou, Q., Stone, S. B., Busse, J. W., Ravindran, N. C., Walter, S. D., Stringer, B., Cook, D. J., Walter, S. D., Sullivan, T., Berwanger, O., Bhandari, M., Banglawala, S., Lavis, J. N., Petrisor, B., Schunemann, H., Walsh, K.,

Bhatnagar, N., Guyatt, G. H., & Burns, K. E. (2009). Quality of care in for-profit and not-for-profit nursing homes: Systematic review and meta-analysis. *BMJ: British Medical Journal*, *339*(7717), 381–384. https://doi.org/10.1136/bmj.b2732

Conti, E. C., Jahn, D. R., Simons, K. V., Edinboro, L. P. C., Jacobs, M. L., Vinson, L., Stahl, S. T., & Van Orden, K. A. (2020). Safety planning to manage suicide risk with older adults: Case examples and recommendations. *Clinical Gerontologist*, *43*(1), 104–109. https://doi.org/10.1080/07317115.2019.1611685

Conwell, Y., Van Orden, K., & Caine, E. D. (2011). Suicide in older adults. *Psychiatric Clinics of North America*, *34*(2), 451–468, ix. https://doi.org/10.1016/j.psc.2011.02.002

Dubljanin Raspopovic, E., Maric, N., Nedeljkovic, U., Ilic, N., Tomanovic Vujadinovic, S., & Bumbasirevic, M. (2014). Do depressive symptoms on hospital admission impact early functional outcome in elderly patients with hip fracture? *Psychogeriatrics*, *14*(2), 118–123. https://doi.org/10.1111/psyg.12049

Ghose, S. S., Williams, L. S., & Swindle, R. W. (2005). Depression and other mental health diagnoses after stroke increase inpatient and outpatient medical utilization three years poststroke. *Medical Care*, *43*(12), 1259–1264. https://doi.org/10.1097/01.mlr.0000185711.50480.13

Gilissen, J., Pivodic, L., Wendrich-van Dael, A., Cools, W., Vander Stichele, R., Van den Block, L., Deliens, L., & Gastmans, C. (2020). Nurses' self-efficacy, rather than their knowledge, is associated with their engagement in advance care planning in nursing homes: A survey study. *Palliative Medicine*, *34*(7), 917–924. https://doi.org/10.1177/0269216320916158

Grabowski, D. C., Aschbrenner, K. A., Feng, Z., & Mor, V. (2009). Mental illness in nursing homes: Variations across States. *Health Affairs*, *28*(3), 689–700. https://doi.org/10.1377/hlthaff.28.3.689

Grabowski, D. C., Aschbrenner, K. A., Rome, V. F., & Bartels, S. J. (2010). Quality of mental health care for nursing home residents: A literature review. *Medical Care Research and Review*, *67*(6), 627–656. https://doi.org/10.1177/1077558710362538

Harrington, C., Olney, B., Carrillo, H., & Kang., T. (2012). Nurse staffing and deficiencies in the largest for-profit chains and chains owned by private equity companies. *Health Services Research*, *47*(1), 106–128. https://doi.org/10.1111/j.1475-6773.2011.01311.x

Harris-Kojetin, L., Sengupta, M., Lendon, J. P., Rome, V., Valverde, R., & Caffrey, C. (2019). Long-term care providers and services users in the United States, 2015-2016. *Vital Health Statistics*, *3*(43), 11. Retrieved https://www.cdc.gov/nchs/nsltcp/nsltcp_reports.htm

Jester, D. J., Hyer, K., Bowblis, J. R., & Meeks, S. (2020). Quality concerns in nursing homes that serve large proportions of residents with serious mental illness. *The Gerontologist*, *60*(7), 1312–1321. https://doi.org/10.1093/geront/gnaa044

Konetzka, R. T., Grabowski, D. C., Perraillon, M. C., & Werner, R. M. (2015). Nursing home 5-star rating system exacerbates disparities in quality, by payer source. *Health Affairs*, *34*(5), 819–827. https://doi.org/10.1377/hlthaff.2014.1084

Lee, S. J., Osteen, P. J., & Frey, J. J. (2016). Predicting changes in behavioral health professionals' clinical practice skills for recognizing and responding to suicide risk. *Journal of the Society for Social Work and Research*, *7*(1), 23–41. https://doi.org/10.1086/685037

Ludwin, B. M., & Meeks, S. (2018). Psychological factors related to nurses' intentions to initiate an antipsychotic or psychosocial intervention with nursing home residents. *Geriatric Nursing*, *39*(5), 584–592. https://doi.org/10.1016/j.gerinurse.2018.04.005

Luoma, J. B., Martin, C. E., & Pearson, J. L. (2002). Contact with mental health and primary care providers before suicide: A review of the evidence. *American Journal of Psychiatry*, *159*(6), 909–916. https://doi.org/10.1176/appi.ajp.159.6.909

McCarthy, J. F., Szymanski, B. R., Karlin, B. E., & Katz, I. R. (2013). Suicide mortality following nursing home discharge in the Department of Veterans Affairs health system. *American Journal of Public Health*, *103*(12), 2261–2266. https://doi.org/10.2105/ajph.2013.301292

Mezuk, B., Ko, T. M., Kalesnikava, V. A., & Jurgens, D. (2019). Suicide among older adults living in or transitioning to residential long-term care, 2003 to 2015. *JAMA Network Open*, *2* (6), e195627. https://doi.org/10.1001/jamanetworkopen.2019.5627

Mezuk, B., Lohman, M., Leslie, M., & Powell, V. (2015). Suicide risk in nursing homes and assisted living facilities: 2003-2011. *American Journal of Public Health*, *105*(7), 1495–1502. https://doi.org/10.2105/AJPH.2015.302573

Mitchell, S. M., Taylor, N. J., Jahn, D. R., Roush, J. F., Brown, S. L., Ries, R., & Quinnett, P. (2020). Suicide-related training, self-efficacy, and mental health care providers' reactions toward suicidal individuals. *Crisis*, *41*(5), 359–366. https://doi.org/10.1027/0227-5910/a000647

National Academies of Sciences, Engineering, and Medicine. (2020). *Social Isolation and loneliness in older adults: Opportunities for the health care system*. The National Academies Press.

National Association of Social Workers. (2003). *NASW standards for social work services in long-term care facilities*. Retrieved: https://www.socialworkers.org/LinkClick.aspx?fileticket=cwW7lzBfYxg%3D&portalid=0s

Orth, J., Li, Y., Simning, A., & Temkin-Greener, H. (2019). Providing behavioral health services in nursing homes is difficult: Findings From a national survey. *Journal of the American Geriatrics Society*, *67*(8), 1713–1717. https://doi.org/10.1111/jgs.16017

Preadmission Screening and Resident Review (PASRR) Technical Assistance Center. (2019). *2019 PASRR National Report: A Review of Preadmission Screening and Resident Review (PASRR) Programs* Retrieved Online: https://23c2beb0-a2ae-4e75-aa9d-4b9d2de03e73.filesusr.com/ugd/d693e6_a6b0cad5964e488a8758d04b3fb1ad17.pdf

Raue, P. J., McGovern, A. R., Kiosses, D. N., & Sirey, J. A. (2017). Advances in psychotherapy for depressed older adults. *Current Psychiatry Reports*, *19*(9), 57. https://doi.org/10.1007/s11920-017-0812-8

Roberts, A. R., & Bowblis, J. R. (2017). Who hires social workers? Structural and contextual determinants of social service staffing in nursing homes. *Health & Social Work*, *42*(1), 15–23. https://doi.org/10.1093/hsw/hlw058

Roberts, A. R., Smith, A. C., & Bowblis, J. R. (2019). *Impact of social service staffing on nursing home quality and resident outcomes*. Scripps Gerontology Center. https://sc.lib.miamioh.edu/bitstream/handle/2374.MIA/6345/Roberts-3-2019-Impact-Social-Service-Staffing-NH-Quality.pdf

Roberts, A. R., Smith, A. C., & Bowblis, J. R. (2020). Nursing home social services and post-acute care: Does more qualified staff improve behavioral symptoms and reduce anti-psychotic drug use? *Journal of the American Medical Directors Association*, *21*(3), 388–394. https://doi.org/10.1016/j.jamda.2019.07.024

Saliba, D., DiFilippo, S., Edelen, M. O., Kroenke, K., Buchanan, J., & Streim, J. (2012). Testing the PHQ-9 interview and observational versions (PHQ-9 OV) for MDS 3.0. *Journal of the American Medical Directors Association*, *13*(7), 618–625. https://doi.org/10.1016/j.jamda.2012.06.003

Seitz, D., Purandare, N., & Conn, D. (2010). Prevalence of psychiatric disorders among older adults in long-term care homes: A systematic review. *International Psychogeriatrics*, *22*(7), 1025–1039. https://doi.org/10.1017/S1041610210000608

Sexton, M., & Orchard, C. (2016). Understanding healthcare professionals' self-efficacy to resolve interprofessional conflict. *Journal of Interprofessional Care*, *30*(3), 316–323. https://doi.org/10.3109/13561820.2016.1147021

Simons, K., Van Orden, K., Conner, K. R., & Bagge, C. (2019). Age differences in suicide risk screening and management prior to suicide attempts. *The American Journal of Geriatric Psychiatry, 27*(6), 604–608. https://doi.org/10.1016/j.jagp.2019.01.017

Stanley, B., Brown, G. K., Brenner, L. A., Galfalvy, H. C., Currier, G. W., Knox, K. L., Chaudhury, S. R., Bush, A. L., & Green, K. L. (2018). Comparison of the safety planning intervention with follow-up vs usual care of suicidal patients treated in the emergency department. *JAMA Psychiatry, 75*(9), 894–900. https://doi.org/10.1001/jamapsychiatry.2018.1776

Szanto, K., Lenze, E. J., Waern, M., Duberstein, P., Bruce, M. L., Epstein-Lubow, G., & Conwell, Y. (2013). Research to reduce the suicide rate among older adults: Methodology roadblocks and promising paradigms. *Psychiatric Services, 64*(6), 586–589. https://doi.org/10.1176/appi.ps.003582012

Temkin-Greener, H., Orth, J., Conwell, Y., & Li, Y. (2020). Suicidal Ideation in US nursing homes: Association with individual and facility factors. *The American Journal of Geriatric Psychiatry, 28*(3), 288–298. https://doi.org/10.1016/j.jagp.2019.12.011

Van Orden, K., & Conwell, Y. (2011). Suicides in late life. *Current Psychiatry Reports, 13*(3), 234–241. https://doi.org/10.1007/s11920-011-0193-3

Van Orden, K. A., Bower, E., Lutz, J., Silva, C., Gallegos, A. M., Podgorski, C. A., Santos, E. J., & Conwell, Y. (2020). Strategies to promote social connections among older adults during 'social distancing' restrictions. *The American Journal of Geriatric Psychiatry.* https://doi.org/10.1016/j.jagp.2020.05.004

Vongxaiburana, E., Thomas, K. S., Frahm, K. A., & Hyer, K. (2011). The social worker in interdisciplinary care planning. *Clinical Gerontologist, 34*(5), 367–378. https://doi.org/10.1080/07317115.2011.588540

Watt, J., Tricco, A. C., Talbot-Hamon, C., Pham, B., Rios, P., Grudniewicz, A., Wong, C., Sinclair, D., & Straus, S. E. (2018). Identifying older adults at risk of harm following elective surgery: A systematic review and meta-analysis. *BMC Medicine, 16*(1), 2. https://doi.org/10.1186/s12916-017-0986-2

Werner, R. M., & Konetzka, R. T. (2018). Trends in post-acute care use among medicare beneficiaries: 2000 to 2015. *JAMA, 319*(15), 1616–1617. https://doi.org/10.1001/jama.2018.2408

More Evidence that Federal Regulations Perpetuate Unrealistic Nursing Home Social Services Staffing Ratios

Mercedes Bern-Klug ⓘ, Kara A. Carter, and Yi Wang

What guides quality psychosocial care in nursing homes? By law, people receiving care in Medicare or Medicaid certified nursing facilities (in this manuscript referred to as nursing homes) are required to have ready access to psychosocial care. Psychosocial issues are those related to the psychological, spiritual, interpersonal, and societal aspects of living (Werth & Blevins, 2006). Residents' psychosocial needs are to be assessed and documented within 48 hours of admission and addressed throughout their nursing home stay (CMS State Operations Manual, 2017, section 483.21). Examples of resident psychosocial issues include dealing with multiple and compounding losses including loss of possessions, health and functional abilities, dignity and privacy, important relationships, role in the community; as well as crisis management; recovering from disrupted relationships; end-of-life decision-making; and advance care planning. Good psychosocial assessment also identifies and builds on residents' psychosocial strengths by supporting them in finding meaning in daily routines; connecting with people and organizations that encourage and support personal growth; and facilitating opportunities to express creativity (Bern-Klug, 2010).

In many nursing homes it is the social worker's responsibility to anticipate and assess residents' psychosocial needs and strengths, and then develop an appropriate care plan. Yet not all nursing homes employ a social worker. The purpose of this article is to draw attention to the disconnect between the federal regulations that hold certified nursing homes responsible for residents' psychosocial needs and the insufficient regulatory standards for both the number and the qualifications of the social work staff whose job it is to document and develop care plans to address psychosocial needs. Although this paper begins by discussing CMS requirements for social work qualifications, our goal here is to report empirical findings related to nursing home social services staffing ratios.

The Federal Role in Nursing Home Regulations

The passage of Medicare and Medicaid in the mid 1960's and their associated coverage of services in nursing homes cemented the federal government's regulatory role regarding the operation of the nursing home industry. In order to be eligible to receive payments from the Medicare and/or Medicaid programs, a nursing home must be certified as meeting the Center for Medicare and Medicaid Services (CMS) requirements. These requirements hold nursing homes responsible for assessing the physical, mental, and psychosocial needs of residents and using assessment data to develop and deliver an individualized plan of care for each resident (Code of Federal Regulations, 2020). Social workers and other members of the social services department typically lead the nursing home's efforts in assessing and addressing resident psychosocial issues. In fact, in a nationally representative sample of nursing home social services directors, 96% reported their department was usually or always involved in developing individualized care plans addressing resident psychosocial needs (Bern-Klug & Cordes, 2021).

Table 1 provides examples of medically related social services listed in the CMS State Operations Manual. Among other functions, social workers screen residents for mental health concerns, address emotional issues, assist with interpersonal conflicts, support residents and families with decision-making, and facilitate transitions between care settings such as hospitals, hospice, or back home as well as provide medically related social services. Staff also use non-pharmacological approaches in working with residents with dementia who may be experiencing behavioral challenges and provide or arrange for counseling services. These services require skill and can impact the experience of living and dying in a nursing home.

As important as the social work role is to the quality of life of nursing home residents, the literature regarding nursing home social work staffing ratios is sparse and the relevant federal regulations are thin. In Medicare and Medicaid certified nursing homes, social work staffing issues are two-fold: 1) who qualifies to be a nursing home social worker; 2) how many social workers a nursing home must employ.

The paper has three aims: 1) document the number of residents that social services directors report one full-time staff person can serve; 2) compare that number to actual social services staffing ratios; and 3) report the characteristics of nursing homes related to social services staffing ratios. In this paper the term, "social services director" refers to the lead staff person in the social services department, who may or may not have earned a social work degree.

Table 1. CMS State Operations Manual: Medically-Related Social Services in Certified Nursing Homes.

§483.40(d) The facility must provide medically-related social services to attain or maintain the highest practicable physical, mental and psychosocial well-being of each resident.

INTENT §483.40(d)

To assure that sufficient and appropriate social services are provided to meet the resident's needs.

DEFINITIONS §483.40(d)

Definitions are provided to clarify terminology related to behavioral health services and the attainment or maintenance of a resident's highest practicable well-being.

"Medically-related social services" means services provided by the facility's staff to assist residents in attaining or maintaining their mental and psychosocial health.

GUIDANCE §483.40(d)

All facilities are required to provide medically-related social services for each resident. Facilities must identify the need for medically-related social services and ensure that these services are provided. It is not required that a qualified social worker necessarily provide all of these services, except as required by State law.

If there are concerns about requirements involving qualified social workers, refer to §483.70(p) (F850), Social worker.

Examples of medically-related social services include, but are not limited to the following:
• Advocating for residents and assisting them in the assertion of their rights within the facility in accordance with §483.10, Resident Rights, §483.12, Freedom from Abuse, Neglect, and Exploitation, §483.15, Transitions of Care, §483.20, Resident Assessments (PASARR), and §483.21, Comprehensive Person-Centered Care Planning;
• Assisting residents in voicing and obtaining resolution to grievances about treatment, living conditions, visitation rights, and accommodation of needs;
• Assisting or arranging for a resident's communication of needs through the resident's primary method of communication or in a language that the resident understands;
• Making arrangements for obtaining items, such as clothing and personal items;
• Assisting with informing and educating residents, their family, and/or representative(s) about health care options and ramifications;
• Making referrals and obtaining needed services from outside entities (e.g., talking books, absentee ballots, community wheelchair transportation);
• Assisting residents with financial and legal matters (e.g., applying for pensions, referrals to lawyers, referrals to funeral homes for preplanning arrangements);
• Transitions of care services (e.g., assisting the resident with identifying community placement options and completion of the application process, arranging intake for home care services for residents returning home, assisting with transfer arrangements to other facilities);
• Providing or arranging for needed mental and psychosocial counseling services;
• Identifying and seeking ways to support residents' individual needs through the assessment and care planning process;
• Encouraging staff to maintain or enhance each resident's dignity in recognition of each resident's individuality;
• Assisting residents with advance care planning, including but not limited to completion of advance directives (For additional information pertaining to advance directives, refer to §483.10(g)(12) (F578)), Advance Directives);
• Identifying and promoting individualized, non-pharmacological approaches to care that meet the mental and psychosocial needs of each resident; and
• Meeting the needs of residents who are grieving from losses and coping with stressful events.

Situations in which the facility should provide social services or obtain needed services from outside entities include, but are not limited to the following:
• Lack of an effective family or community support system or legal representative;
• Expressions or indications of distress that affect the resident's mental and psychosocial well-being, resulting from depression, chronic diseases (e.g., Alzheimer's disease and other dementia related diseases, schizophrenia, multiple sclerosis), difficulty with personal interaction and socialization skills, and resident to resident altercations;
• Abuse of any kind (e.g., alcohol or other drugs, physical, psychological, sexual, neglect, exploitation);
• Difficulty coping with change or loss (e.g., change in living arrangement, change in condition or functional ability, loss of meaningful employment or activities, loss of a loved one); and
• Need for emotional support.

Source: CMS (2017) State Operations Manual, Appendix PP – Guidance to surveyors for long-term care facilities. https://www.cms.gov/Medicare/Provider-Enrollment-and-Certification/GuidanceforLawsAndRegulations/Downloads/Appendix-PP-State-Operations-Manual.pdf

Background

Federal Regulations Related to Who is Qualified to be a Nursing Home Social Worker

When it comes to determining who is qualified for employment as a social worker in a nursing home, federal regulations (i.e., CMS regulations) deviate from professional standards developed by the National Association of Social Workers (NASW) and state laws because CMS does not require a degree in social work for nursing home social work employment. CMS rules state:

> A qualified social worker is: (1) An individual with a minimum of a bachelor's degree in social work or a bachelor's degree in a human services field including, but not limited to, sociology, gerontology, special education, rehabilitation counseling, and psychology; and (2) One year of supervised social work experience in a health care setting working directly with individuals.

> Code of Federal Regulations (2020). Title 42 (Public Health), chapter IV, subchapter G, Part 483-subpart B Section 483.70 (Administration).

The CMS definition of a qualified social worker is not consistent with NASW professional standards, despite CMS's own requirement that nursing homes hire staff whose qualifications comply with professional standards. The Code of Federal Regulations states that services provided by or arranged by certified nursing homes for residents, must:

(i) Meet professional standards of quality.
(ii) Be provided by qualified persons in accordance with each resident's written plan of care.
(iii) Be culturally competent and trauma informed.

> Code of Federal Regulations (2020) section 483.21

The National Association of Social Workers' (NASW) has two levels of standards for social work services in long-term care one for social workers and one for social work directors. The NASW qualifications to be a nursing home social worker are having a minimum of a Bachelor of Social Work degree from a program accredited by the Council on Social Work Education (CSWE), two years postgraduate experience in a long-term care or related setting, and meeting state licensure qualifications. The NASW defines a social work *director* as preferably holding a Master of Social Work degree (NASW National Association of Social Workers, 2003). The NASW standards do not indicate what is an appropriate social work staffing ratio in nursing homes.

In direct opposition to national professional standards, which require a social work degree from a program accredited by the Council on Social Work Education (CSWE), in nursing homes CMS allows people to serve as "qualified social workers" without a college degree in social work. While we recognize the important work that nonsocial workers are engaged in, we note that social services staff members with a degree in sociology or gerontology (allowed by federal regulations) are not required to complete an internship, nor demonstrate basic clinical interpersonal skills, nor basic competency in how to intervene in systems change at the individual, family, small group, organizational, and community levels. (Please see American Sociology Association, 2014 for information about coursework and preparation). It is at odds with state title protection laws and confusing to residents, families, staff members, and the community to call a person who has not earned a degree in social work, a "qualified" social worker.

As shown in Table 2, in no other health setting receiving CMS funds, does a "qualified social worker" include a person who has not graduated from an accredited social work program. CMS accepts profession standards for the operationalization of physicians, pharmacists, nurses, dietitians, and physical therapists, but not social workers in nursing homes.

Federal Regulations Related to Social Work Staffing Ratios: The 120 Rule

Besides CMS's unique operationalization of a "qualified social worker" in the nursing home setting, regulations regarding the practice of nursing home social work are limited in another important way. While CMS holds all certified nursing homes responsible for addressing psychosocial issues of all residents, CMS requires nursing homes to employ one full-time "qualified social worker" *only* if the nursing home has more than 120 beds (Code of Federal Regulations, 2020). Two-thirds of the nursing homes in the United States have fewer than 120 beds (Harris-Kojetin et al., 2019). Facilities with 120 or fewer beds can hire a part-time person or contract with an agency to provide psychosocial care and social services. If a nursing home with 120 or fewer beds decides to hire a social services staff person, federal guidelines have *no* educational requirements for these staff members. Furthermore, the federal government requires no nursing home, regardless of the number of beds, to hire more than one federally "qualified social worker."

The "120-bed rule" was included in the Nursing Home Reform Act which was part of the landmark OBRA 1987 (PL-100-103) legislation. According to Dr. Roberta Greene (social work scholar who was representing NASW at a meeting on Capitol Hill to discuss nursing home regulations in the late 1980s), the number was determined after an aide in Senator George Mitchell's (Maine) office called a constituent during a planning meeting attended by Dr. Greene and asked the constituent for advice on an appropriate number. The constituent suggested that no nursing home with 120 or fewer beds should be required to employ a full-time social worker (personal communication, 2018). At the time no nursing home in Maine had more than 120 beds.

Table 2. Requirements for Social Work Professionals in Medicare and/or Medicaid Certified Health Facilities as Reported in Title 42 of the Code of Federal Regulations (CFR).

Facility type	Social work qualifications
Nursing homes Nursing facilities and skilled nursing facilities	(p) *Social worker.* Any facility with more than 120 beds must employ a qualified social worker on a full-time basis. A qualified social worker is: (1) An individual with a minimum of a bachelor's degree in social work or a bachelor's degree in a human services field including, but not limited to, sociology, gerontology, special education, rehabilitation counseling, and psychology; and (2) One year of supervised social work experience in a health care setting working directly with individuals. 42CFR483.70
Intermediate Care Facilities for Individuals with Intellectual Disabilities	(5) Professional program staff must be licensed, certified, or registered, as applicable, to provide professional services by the State in which he or she practices. Those professional program staff who do not fall under the jurisdiction of State licensure, certification, or registration requirements, specified in §483.410(b), must meet the following qualifications: (includes other as well as) (vi) To be designated as a social worker, an individual must – (A) Hold a graduate degree from a school of social work accredited or approved by the Council on Social Work Education or another comparable body; or (B) Hold a Bachelor of Social Work degree from a college or university accredited or approved by the Council on Social Work Education or another comparable body. 42CFR483.430
Hospice	(3) *Social worker.* A person who – (i)(A) Has a Master of Social Work (MSW) degree from a school of social work accredited by the Council on Social Work Education; or (B) Has a baccalaureate degree in social work from an institution accredited by the Council on Social Work Education; or a baccalaureate degree in psychology, sociology, or other field related to social work and is supervised by an MSW as described in paragraph (b)(3)(i)(A) of this section; and (ii) Has 1 year of social work experience in a healthcare setting; or (iii) Has a baccalaureate degree from a school of social work accredited by the Council on Social Work Education, is employed by the hospice before December 2, 2008, and is not required to be supervised by an MSW. 42CFR 418.114
Hospital	(5) Any discharge planning evaluation or discharge plan required under this paragraph must be developed by, or under the supervision of, a registered nurse, social worker, or other appropriately qualified personnel. 42CFR482.43
Transplant Center	(d) Standard: Social services. The transplant center must make social services available, furnished by qualified social workers, to transplant patients, living donors, and their families. A qualified social worker is an individual who meets licensing requirements in the State in which he or she practices; and (1) Completed a course of study with specialization in clinical practice and holds a master's degree from a graduate school of social work accredited by the Council on Social Work Education; or (2) Is working as a social worker in a transplant center as of the effective date of this final rule and has served for at least 2 years as a social worker, 1 year of which was in a transplantation program, and has established a consultative relationship with a social worker who is qualified under (d)(1) of this paragraph. 42 CFR 482.94(d)

(*Continued*)

Table 2. (Continued).

Facility type	Social work qualifications
Home Health	(3) Medical social services are provided under the supervision of a social worker that meets the requirements of §484.115(m). 42CFR484.75 And: (l) *Standard: Social Work Assistant.* A person who provides services under the supervision of a qualified social worker and: (1) Has a baccalaureate degree in social work, psychology, sociology, or other field related to social work, and has had at least 1 year of social work experience in a health care setting; or (2) Has 2 years of appropriate experience as a social work assistant, and has achieved a satisfactory grade on a proficiency examination conducted, approved, or sponsored by the U.S. Public Health Service, except that the determinations of proficiency do not apply with respect to persons initially licensed by a state or seeking initial qualification as a social work assistant after December 31, 1977. (m) *Standard: Social worker.* A person who has a master's or doctoral degree from a school of social work accredited by the Council on Social Work Education, and has 1 year of social work experience in a health care setting. 42CFR484.115
Comprehensive Outpatient Rehabilitation Facility	(l) A *social worker* must – (1) Be licensed by the State in which practicing, if applicable; (2) Hold at least a bachelor's degree from a school accredited or approved by the Council on Social Work Education; and (3) Have 1 year of social work experience in a health care setting. 42CFR485.70
End-Stage Renal Disease Facilities	(d) *Standard: Social worker.* The facility must have a social worker who – (1) Holds a master's degree in social work with a specialization in clinical practice from a school of social work accredited by the Council on Social Work Education; or (2) Has served at least 2 years as a social worker, 1 year of which was in a dialysis unit or transplantation program prior to September 1, 1976, and has established a consultative relationship with a social worker who qualifies under §494.140(d)(1). 42CFR494.140
Psychiatry Hospital	(f) *Standard: Social services.* There must be a director of social services who monitors and evaluates the quality and appropriateness of social services furnished. The services must be furnished in accordance with accepted standards of practice and established policies and procedures. (1) The director of the social work department or service must have a master's degree from an accredited school of social work or must be qualified by education and experience in the social services needs of the mentally ill. If the director does not hold a masters degree in social work, at least one staff member must have this qualification. (2) Social service staff responsibilities must include, but are not limited to, participating in discharge planning, arranging for follow-up care, and developing mechanisms for exchange of appropriate, information with sources outside the hospital. 42CFR482.62
Rural Health Clinic and Federally Qualified Health Center	(6) A physician, nurse practitioner, physician assistant, certified nurse-midwife, clinical social worker, or clinical psychologist is available to furnish patient care services at all times the clinic or center operates. In addition, for RHCs, a nurse practitioner, physician assistant, or certified nurse-midwife is available to furnish patient care services at least 50% of the time the RHC operates. 42CFR491.8

Note: In Veterans Affairs (VA) nursing homes, a social worker is a person with a master's degree in social work. https://www.socialwork.va.gov/

Back in 1987 when the "120 rule" was established, most residents in nursing homes were there to receive long-term care for assistance with activities of daily living. At the time, some nursing homes were just beginning to modify their business strategy in response to the major changes in Medicare laws that were enacted in 1983, specifically the introduction of a new prospective payment system for hospitals. The prospective payment plan provided a financial incentive for hospitals to discharge patients when they no longer required hospital-level care (Altman, 2012). This often meant the patient was not sick enough to stay in the hospital and yet not well enough to go home and so was discharged to a nursing home to receive post-acute care. Sometimes referred to as sub-acute other times as post-acute, the level of care is not as intense as hospital-level care and yet skilled nursing and/or rehabilitation care is required. When the 120-bed rule was first enacted, nursing homes were providing long-term care almost exclusively, and most of that care was paid for by Medicaid. As mentioned earlier, currently, most nursing homes provide post-acute care as well as long-term care, and the post-acute care is paid by Medicare at a rate profitable to nursing homes (MedPAC (Medicare Payment Advisory Commission), 2020).

By 2016 almost all (97.5%) certified nursing homes were eligible to receive Medicare funding for the provision of post-acute care and 95% were eligible to receive both Medicare and Medicaid funding (Harris-Kojetin et al., 2019). Nursing homes have a financial incentive to admit people with post-acute care needs covered by Medicare. The daily Medicare rate for residents receiving post-acute care is higher than the Medicaid rate for the provision of long-term care, and the Medicare profit margins are higher too, " . . . Medicare reimbursements remain the most prized source of revenue for nursing facility operators, as they come in several hundreds of dollars per day higher than rates from Medicare Advantage plans and Medicaid" (Spanko, 2020). MedPAC (Medicare Payment Advisory Commission) (2020) reports the Medicare margins for skilled nursing facilities amounted to 10% in 2018, down from 14% in 2012 and 21% in 2011 (MedPAC (Medicare Payment Advisory Commission), 2020, p. 101). The reimbursement changes and challenges facing nursing homes are an important part of the context of care provision.

Fashaw et al. (2020) looked back thirty years to the passage of the Nursing Home Reform Act of 1987 and documented changes in the type of care provided and the characteristics of the people receiving care in U.S. nursing homes. They reported that compared to decades ago, more people are being admitted directly from the hospital for a short stay of post-acute care and there is a dramatic increase in the number of residents with serious mental illness. They also documented that a high proportion of long-stay residents are people with dementia. While 80 is the average age of residents (Fashaw et al., 2020, p. 235), a growing proportion – now 17% – have not yet reached age 65 (Harris-Kojetin et al., 2019, p. 20). Hay and Chaudhury (2015) describe some of the ways psychosocial needs of younger nursing home residents can differ from older residents.

The change over the past decades from nursing homes providing mostly long-term care to providing post-acute care has implications for the type of social work services needed. Post-acute social work care involves working with people who have just completed a hospital stay, often because of an unexpected serious medical crisis such as broken hip or a stroke. The change in functional ability is often swift and profound and yet with rehabilitation, the person is expected to recover function. Restorative care is an important component of post-acute services (CMS, 2017). There are more frequent requirements for staff to document the services provided compared with residents receiving long-term care (CMS, 2017). Because the length of stay is shorter for people receiving post-acute care than for people receiving long-term care, there is more turn-over and consequently the post-acute social work role has a heavy emphasis on discharge planning. Heavy turnover among people receiving post-acute care means more time from social work staff in helping individuals and families adjust to the nursing home and adjust to leaving the nursing home, often with supportive community services that the social worker helps to arrange.

On the other hand, residents admitted for long-term care generally remain for months or years – much longer than post-acute residents, and for some the nursing home becomes their home. Residents receiving long-term care are often dealing with gradual and progressive changes due to advancing chronic illnesses. They may be facing psychosocial issues related to grief and loss, meaning making, medical decision-making, advance care planning, and related issues related to living with advancing and chronic illnesses.

The different social work needs of people receiving post-acute care versus long-term care should be factored in when considering social work staffing ratios. Despite the steady and dramatic growth in post-acute care, and therefore the need for more intensive medically related social services over the past 40 years, CMS has not updated regulations related to the number of residents one social worker can serve. To this day, only nursing homes with more than 120 beds are required to employ one (and only one) full-time social worker, regardless of the number of residents receiving post-acute care.

What is a realistic staffing ratio according to the people working in the role? In stark contrast to the "120-bed rule," the majority of respondents in a 2006 nationally representative study of nursing home social services directors reported that one full-time social services staff member could meet the psychosocial care needs of fewer than 60 long-term care residents *or* fewer than 20 post-acute residents (Bern-Klug et al., 2010). We update those figures in this paper.

Staffing Ratios Impact Outcomes

Most of the research examining the impact of staffing ratios on resident outcomes looks at nursing ratios. Considerable literature (Castle, 2008; Castle & Banaszak-Holl, 2003; CMS, 2020; Geng et al., 2019; Harrington et al., 2000) documents that as staff availability increases, so does the quality of care. Nursing homes with fewer residents per nursing staff member have higher quality of resident care and fewer deficiencies (Harrington et al., 2000). The literature also continues to document that the quality of care in nursing homes varies by facility ownership type (Aaronson et al., 1994; Bonifas, 2011; Harrington et al., 2000; Hillmer et al., 2005; Roberts & Bowblis, 2017). Not-for-profit and government operated nursing homes tend to have higher quality ratings, fewer deficiencies, and overall, more resident-favorable (fewer residents per staff member) staffing ratios than for-profit facilities.

Only a few studies have considered staffing issues in nursing homes among non-nursing staff. Castle and Banaszak-Holl (2003) document a strong positive relationship between nursing home administrative staffing hours and resident outcomes and quality of care. Harrington et al. (2000) examined both resident quality of care and quality of life outcomes in relationship to both nursing and other staff (including social services) in nursing homes. They found that higher numbers of residents per nursing staff was related to lower quality of care outcomes, and higher numbers of residents per other staff resulted in lower resident quality of life outcomes.

Methods

Data for this study come from the 2019 National Nursing Home Social Services Directors Study, administered at the University of Iowa School of Social Work with IRB approval and with funding from the RRF Foundation for Aging.

Participants

Findings reported in this paper are from a nationally representative sample of 837 nursing home social services directors, most of whom reported their gender as female (91%) and their race as white (87%). In terms of age, 28% were 18–34 years of age, 47% were 35–54 years of age, and 25% were ages 55 or older. Respondents reported a wide variety of educational attainment. One in ten reported a high school degree as their highest level of education, six percent reported an associate's degree as their highest level of education, and 50% a bachelor's degree (with 30% of the sample with a Bachelor of Social Work, BSW). About one-third (35%) of respondents reported their highest level of education at the master's level, most of whom had earned a master's degree in social work (MSW) (28% of the sample). Almost half (46%) of the sample reported holding a state license or certification in social work, including people who had not earned a degree in social work (allowed in some states under limited circumstances). More information about respondent characteristics can be found at Bern-Klug, et al., 2021.

Sampling Frame

The CMS Nursing Home Compare publicly available datafile was used as the sampling frame. The datafile contained information about the 15,578 Medicare and/or Medicaid certified nursing homes as of December 2018. Using the random sampling function in SPSS v25, we selected 3,650 nursing homes and downloaded their address, phone number, and basic characteristics such as the number of beds. Phone calls were attempted to the nursing homes in the sample to determine the presence of at least one social services staff person who worked at least part time and to secure that staff person's e-mail. An invitation was mailed (electronically or by ground) addressed to the social services director. In all, 3,065 invitations were sent (indicating that most nursing homes (84%) – even those with fewer than 120 beds – do employ at least one person at least part-time in social services). The response rate was 30%; 924 surveys were returned. Data from 837 of the 924 respondents are used in this paper. More information about the sampling can be found at Bern-Klug, et al., 2021.

Survey Instrument and Data

The primary purpose of the original study was to collect data describing the characteristics and functions of social services departments and the training needs of social services directors. The questionnaire was adapted from a similar study undertaken in 2006 (Bern-Klug et al., 2009). A national advisory committee of nursing home social work scholars, practitioners, and advocates was consulted on the adaptations, and the questionnaire was pilot tested with employed nursing home social services staff members. The final questionnaire contained 185 items related to departmental responsibilities, training needs, barriers to providing psychosocial care, description of work conditions, and job satisfaction was developed and pilot tested. The questions used to develop this manuscript are described in detail below. To reduce respondent burden, variables describing characteristics of the nursing home (number of beds, profit status, region of the country, metro status, and quality rating) from the publicly available CMS nursing home compare datafile (https://data.cms.gov/provider-data/topics/nursing-homes) were downloaded and were merged with data supplied by respondents.

Variables

Opinions on appropriate staffing ratios. In two separate questions, respondents were asked their opinion about staffing ratios. One question asked about long-term care residents and the other about post-acute residents, as reported below:

> "In your opinion, about how many long-term care residents can one full-time social services staff person handle in terms of assessing psychosocial needs, care planning and providing/coordinating psychosocial care delivery? (Assuming caring only for LTC residents; no responsibility for short-term skilled/rehab/post/sub-acute care residents?) One full-time social services staff per _____ LTC residents."

Response categories were less than 30; 30–59; 60–89; 90–119, 120–140; more than 140. The next question substituted long-term care residents with "short-term skilled/rehab/post/sub-acute care patients." The response categories for this question included: less than 10; 11–20; 21–29; 30–39; 40–49; 50–59; 60–69; and 70 or more.

Proportion of effort devoted to post-acute residents. We did not have access to data that would indicate the proportion of residents in each nursing home receiving post-acute care paid by Medicare and the proportion receiving long-term care. Without those data, it is not possible to calculate post-acute social services staffing ratios and long-term care social services staffing ratios. We did ask respondents to provide a sense of the amount of the social services' departmental effort devoted to providing care to post-acute residents. We asked: "About what percent of social services staff time is spent on short-term patients (post-acute, sub-acute, rehab, skilled)?" The response categories were: 0%; 1–24%; 25–49%; 50–74%; 75–99%; 100.

Regression analysis dependent variable. Full-time equivalent (FTE) social services staffing ratio is the dependent variable. To determine the actual social services staffing ratio we divided the number of full-time equivalent social services staff hours by the number of beds, and then multiplied by 100 to be able to report the number of social services FTE per 100 beds.

We calculated the number of full-time equivalent staffing hours from responses to two questions. First, we asked how many people worked in the social services department (possible answers: one, two, three, or four or more people). Then we ask the number of hours each social services staff member worked in a typical week: less than 20 hours; 20–34 hours or 35 or more hours, for up to three staff members. FTE was calculated only for nursing homes with three or fewer social services staff members, which amounted to 94% of 924 nursing homes represented in the study. The social services full-time equivalent for each nursing homes was divided by the number of beds. The final number was multiplied by 100 to be able to standardize the social services staffing ratio per 100 beds.

Regression analysis independent variables. Data describing the characteristics of the nursing home came from CMS Nursing Home Compare datafile, available to the public from the medicare.gov website:

"Bed size" is the number of beds in each facility. Two-tail hypothesis is proposed: Bed size is related to the number of residents per social services FTE.

"Quality rating" is calculated and reported by CMS and is one of three measures that factor into the *CMS 5-Star Quality Rating System* (CMS, 2020) and posted on the CMS nursing home compare website. CMS develops a quality rating for each nursing home based on resident assessment data, for example, the percentage of residents whose need for help with activities of daily living increased (CMS, 2020). Quality ratings can range from 1–5, with 5 being the highest quality. We are proposing a one-tail hypothesis: nursing homes with high quality ratings will have fewer residents per social services staff member FTE.

"Ownership Type" reflects the tax status of the nursing home. The CMS datafile listed ten types of ownership, which we recoded into these three: for-profit, government, and nonprofit. We are proposing a one tail hypothesis: For profit nursing homes will have more residents per social services staff FTE compared to government and not-for-profit nursing homes.

"County type" has two levels, metro or non-metro and was determined based on county location of each nursing home, using the USDA's Rural Urban Continuum Code (RUCC) available at https://www.ers.usda.gov/data-products/rural-urban-continuum-codes.aspx. We are proposing a two-tailed hypothesis. County status will be related to number of residents per social services FTE.

"Region" has four levels. The 50 states and District of Columbia were grouped into U.S. Census Bureau categories for regions including: Northeast, South, Midwest, and West. We are proposing a two-tailed hypothesis: Region will be related to the number of residents per social services FTE.

Analysis

Descriptive statistics were used to address the first two study aims (1) document the number of residents that social services directors report one full-time staff member can serve; 2) report the average social services staffing ratio. Linear regression was used to address the third aim, i.e., to report the characteristics of nursing homes related to social services staffing ratios.

For the regression analyses, as a diagnostic step, the normality of the data was assessed. The regression analyses were conducted using Stata version 15. Six outliers were deleted due to extreme values on the dependent variable. The final working sample consisted of 837 nursing homes that had complete information on all the variables in the multivariate regression model.

The average variance inflation factor (VIF) value for our model was 1.8, which is below the "standard" threshold (Johnston et al., 2018), indicating no evidence of harmful multicollinearity. Considering that there may be within-region clustering effects, we also conducted a sensitivity analysis of multilevel modeling. The intraclass correlation coefficient (ICC) for social service staffing ratios in this study was 0.037, indicating that only a small amount (3.7%) of the variability of the dependent variable was accounted for by the inter-region differences. Empirically, the low value of the ICC suggested that we proceed with using single-level analyses (Hox, 2010).

Results

Table 3 reports the characteristics of the nursing homes represented in the study. The number of beds ranged from 18 to 375 with a mean of 98.08. The mean quality rating was 3.96 (out of a possible high of 5). Two-thirds were in metropolitan county and 65% were for profit nursing homes.

Aim 1: When asked how many *long-term care* residents one full-time equivalent social services staff member could handle in terms of psychosocial responsibilities, two-thirds (66%) of the respondents reported less than 60 residents.

When asked how many *short-term* (skilled/rehab/post/sub-acute care) persons one full-time social services staff member could handle, over half (53%) reported 20 or fewer residents, and 75% of the social services directors reported less than 30 residents.

Aim 2: Report the average social services staffing ratio. Social services staffing ranged from 0.27 to 6.67 FTE per 100 residents. The median was 1.49 social services staff per 100 residents and the mean was 1.62 (SD = 0.80). We did not have the data necessary to calculate a separate social service staffing

Table 3. Characteristics of nursing homes (n = 837).

Variables	Mean (SD)/ Freq (%)
Social Services Staff per 100 residents (0.27 ~ 6.67)	1.62 (0.80)
Bed Size (18 ~ 375)	98.08 (45.30)
Quality Rating (1 ~ 5)	3.96 (1.21)
Ownership Type	
For-Profit	541 (64.64)
Government	57 (6.81)
Nonprofit	239 (28.55)
County Type	
Metro County	546 (65.23)
Non-Metro County	291 (34.77)
Regions	
Northeast	120 (14.34)
Midwest	350 (41.82)
South	253 (30.23)
West	114 (13.62)

ratio for post-acute versus long-term care residents. Although we did collect data about the amount of time spent with post-acute resident care needs.

There was wide variation in the proportion of social services staff time devoted to post-acute residents, as reported by the social services director. Seventeen percent of respondents reported less than 24% of staff time spent on post-acute residents. One-quarter of respondents reported that between 25–49% of social services staff time was spent with post-acute residents, and 34% reported between 50 – 74%. Eighteen percent reported 75–99% and two percent of respondents indicated 100% of social services staff time was spent on post-acute residents. Therefore, over half of the respondents reported that at least half of the social services staff time was devoted to providing care to post-acute residents.

Aim 3: Identify characteristics of nursing homes that account for variations in social services staffing ratios. As reported in Table 4, variations in staffing FTE ratio were observed by nursing home ownership status, with nonprofit and government facilities having statistically significantly higher number of FTE social services staff per 100 residents (or said differently, fewer residents per social services staff member). Nonprofit nursing homes generally employed 0.281 more social services FTE in comparison to for-profit nursing homes, and government operated facilities generally employed 0.399 more social services FTE than for-profit facilities.

As reported in Table 4, statistical analysis indicated an inverse relationship between number of beds and staffing. For each one-bed increase in size, facilities saw a *decrease* of 0.008 in social services FTE. The average facility quality rating was 3.96. There was a positive relationship between quality rating and staffing. For each point increase in facility quality rating there was a 0.043 increase in social services FTE.

Holding the effects of the other independent variables constant, social services staffing ratio varied by U.S. region, with the West region reporting the highest social services staff FTE per 100 residents. As reported in Table 4, using the Midwest region as the reference category we found that the Western

Table 4. Results of Regression Model Predicting Social Services Staffing Ratio (n = 837).

Variable	Coef.	S.E.	P	95% CI
Bed Size	−0.0080	0.0006	0.000	−0.009, −0.007
Quality Rating	0.0432	0.020	0.031	0.004, 0.082
Ownership Type (ref. For-Profit)				
Government	0.3994	0.1222	0.001	0.1594, 0.6393
Nonprofit	0.2810	0.0568	0.000	0.1696, 0.3925
Metro (ref. non-metro)	0.1184	0.0500	0.018	0.0202, 0.2166
Region (ref. Midwest)				
Northeast	−0.0347	0.0573	0.544	−0.1472, 0.0777
South	−0.0969	0.0569	0.089	−0.2085, 0.0147
West	0.2199	0.0827	0.008	0.0576, 0.3821
Constant	2.0487	0.1096	0.000	1.8335, 2.2638
R^2	0.2969			

region had 0.220 greater social services FTE than the Midwest. There was no statistical difference between the South and Northeast regions and the Midwest. Nursing homes in metro counties had 0.118 higher social services FTE compared to those in non-metro counties.

Discussion

Federal rules require all Medicare and/or Medicaid certified nursing homes to meet the psychosocial and medically related social services needs of all residents. Only facilities with more than 120 beds are required to employ one full-time federally "qualified social worker" to assess psychosocial concerns and social services needs and provide a care plan for those needs. In this study, we document that despite nursing homes with 120 or fewer beds not being required by the federal government to hire social services staff, most do. This is consistent with federal reports which indicate that 89% of Medicare and/or Medicaid certified nursing homes hire a social services staff member (Harris-Kojetin et al., 2019, p. 10). Our findings indicate social services departments are small, with just over half (54%) employing only one person. Of the nursing homes that do hire social service staff, 94% employ three or fewer full or part-time people.

One of the main findings is that the number of residents one full-time social serivces staff member can meet the needs of is much smaller than the 120 bed rule set by CMS almost 40 years ago. Consistent with what was documented in 2006 (Bern-Klug et al., 2010), we found that the majority of social services directors reported that one full-time social services staff person could assess and meet the psychosocial needs of 60 or fewer long-term care residents *or* 20 or fewer post-acute residents. This is far fewer residents than the CMS regulations requiring only one full-time equivalent social services staff member in facilities with more than 120 beds – regardless of the proportion of post-acute versus long-term care residents. Evidence now from two nationally representative studies of close to 2,000 nursing home social services directors indicates that the federal rules for social services staffing ratios are insufficient.

A second important finding is the actual social services staffing ratio in certified nursing homes. Our data indicate a large standard deviation around the mean ratio of 1.62 social service staff full-time equivalents to 100 residents. This average ratio does not take into account the distribution of residents receiving post-acute versus long-term care.

Over half of the respondents reported that a large proportion of the social services department staff time was devoted to caring for post-acute residents. This is consistent with the distribution of post-acute and long-term care residents reported in a recent federal report stated that 43% of nursing home residents were receiving post-acute care and 57% long-term care (Harris-Kojetin et al., 2019). Therefore, the social services staffing ratio reported above is worse than it appears given that staff can meet the needs of far fewer residents with post-acute needs compared with residents requiring long-term care.

Harris-Kojetin et al. (2019) document that on average, nursing home residents receive five minutes of social work care per day (figure11, p. 13). With so many residents and so few social services staff, it is likely that many resident psychosocial needs are going unassessed and unaddressed. This is exactly what the Office of the Inspector General (OIG) found in their 2003 study of post-acute care residents only (they did not include residents receiving long-term care). The OIG documented many post-acute residents were not receiving adequate psychosocial care, in part due to the inadequacy of the 120-bed rule (Office of the Inspector General, 2003). It is important to address, not just assess resident psychosocial concerns (Bonifas, 2011). Additional evidence comes from social work research scholar, Dr. Robin Bonifas. In her study of nursing homes in Washington state, Bonifas (2008) reported that social services departments with higher caseloads had more difficulty providing effective psychosocial care.

A third finding is that when controlling for the other variables in the regression equation, facility size, quality rating and ownership type accounted for 29.69% of the variance in social services staffing ratio. Our findings indicate that in general, nonprofit and government operated nursing homes have higher social services FTE (fewer residents per social services staff member) than do for-profit facilities. This is congruent with existing literature which examines nursing home ownership type in relationship to nursing home staffing practices (Aaronson et al., 1994; Harrington et al., 2000; Hillmer et al., 2005; Roberts & Bowblis, 2017). Facility size varied widely in our sample, from 18 to 375 beds, with an average of approximately 98 beds. We found that for each one bed increase in facility size there was a related statistically significant *decrease* in social services FTE. This implies that even as facilities serve a greater number of residents, more social services staff are not added to the service provision.

Additionally, there are no federal requirements regarding access to social services (including professional social work services) that take into account the proportion of residents with post-acute needs versus those with long-term care needs. The 2006 findings (Bern-Klug et al., 2010) and the 2019 findings reported here collected directly from social serivces directors clearly documents the need to take residents' needs into account when deciding social services staffing ratios.

CMS requires that all residents receive a comprehensive assessment within 48 hours of admission and a comprehensive care plan based on that assessment be developed by the interdisciplinary team within seven days of completing the assessment. Both the assessment process and the care plan process are required to address psychosocial and medically related social services needs. CMS requires that the interdisciplinary team include the following four members: the attending physician, a registered nurse with responsibility for the resident, a nurse aide with responsibility for the resident, and a member of food and nutrition services staff. CMS does not currently require a social worker on the interdisciplinary care plan team in nursing homes (CMS, SOM, 483.21 2017). Nursing homes are allowed to include additional team members, according to resident needs. It is unclear which of the required four team members is qualified to thoroughly assess and care plan for resident psychosocial and social services needs. For CMS to meet the goals related to developing care plans that address psychosocial and medical related social services needs, we strongly recommend that a social worker be a required member of the interdisciplinary team for all residents. A review of the literature did not reveal any research documenting whether surveyors are checking the qualifications of nursing home social services staff members. We recommend educational and experience qualifications be verified.

Nursing home social services staffing should be reflective of the needs of the population being served and should take into account the proportion of post acute and long-term care residents. Because the federal regulations do not take into account the growing number of post-acute care residents, it is highly likely that residents are at risk of not receiving the care they deserve and social services staff are at risk of being overworked, understaffed, and burnt out. As previous scholars have indicated, social services staffing impacts resident quality of life (Bonifas, 2008; Roberts & Bowblis, 2017; Zhang et al., 2008-2009). Poor staffing practices, guided by inadequate or lax regulations, can negatively impact the daily lives of people receiving care in nursing homes and the people working there. This study provides further evidence that CMS requirements that provide access to psychosocial and medically related social services care for the nation's nursing home residents are inadequate.

Limitations

These findings are from a cross-sectional study with a response rate of 30%. A limitation of this study is that we report one staffing ratio per nursing home, and (because we do not have the data) we do not take into account the proportion of residents receiving post-acute and the proportion receiving long-term care. Also, this study included only one measure of quality of care, and that variable was not directly tied to care provided by social services staff.

Conclusion

This study examined nursing home social services staffing ratios based on primary data collected as part of the National Nursing Home Social Services Director's Survey of 2019 and contributes to the growing literature on nursing home social services. Our data indicate that over half of respondents reported that at least half of the social services staff time was devoted to post-acute residents, meaning that the overall staffing ratio for long-term care residents reported here is even farther away from what social services directors report it should be, in order for them to be able to assess and address residents' psychosocial needs.

Despite the current federal regulations, we believe the evidence is clear that even the best prepared and most highly motivated social worker cannot meet the needs of 120+ residents, a high percentage of whom may be there for post-acute services. Current CMS regulations regarding social services staffing are failing nursing home residents because too few social services staff are being required to meet the needs of both post-acute and long-term care nursing home residents. Furthermore, a separate issue besides the number of staff per resident is the qualifications of the social services staff. CMS regulations are in direct opposition to national professional standards (NASW National Association of Social Workers, 2003). It is important to bear in mind that social workers interact with residents' families as well, further adding to their time commitments, skill needs, and to the amount of emotional labor required to do the job well.

CMS regulations are insufficient to meet the psychosocial and medically related social services needs of the nation's nursing home residents. Just as different levels of nursing (RN, LPN, CNA) are required to meet resident needs, different levels of social work expertise are needed as well. We need professional social workers (i.e., with a social work degree and license) and social work assistants. Social services departments should be led by a licensed social worker and staffed by enough appropriately qualified people to meet resident needs. We recommend one full-time social worker for up to the first 60 long-term care residents, and more social services staff (professional and para-professional) for additional residents. Based on evidence from people doing the work, we recommend one full-time professional social worker for 20 post-acute residents.

Funding

This work was supported by the RRF Foundation for Aging.

ORCID

Mercedes Bern-Klug ⓘ http://orcid.org/0000-0001-6546-6141

References

Aaronson, W. E., Zinn, J. S., & Rosko, M. D. (1994). Do for-profit and not-for-profit nursing homes behave differently? *The Gerontologist*, *34*(6), 775–786. https://doi.org/10.1093/ger ont/34.6.775

Altman, S. H. (2012). The lessons of Medicare's prospective payment system show that the bundled payment program faces challenges. *Health Affairs, 31*(9), 9. https://doi.org/https:// doi.org/https://doi.org/10.1377/hlthaff.2012.0323

American Sociology Association. (2014). *21st century careers with an undergraduate degree in sociology.* https://asa.enoah.com/Store/Career-Publications/BKctl/ViewDetails/SKU/ ASAOE500C14

Bern-Klug, M. (2010). *Transforming palliative care in nursing homes: The social work role.* Columbia University Press.

Bern-Klug, M., & Cordes, E. (2021). Dementia tops training needs of nursing home social services directors; Discharge responsibilities are common core functions of the department. *Journal of Gerontological Social Work*, 1–17. https://doi.org/10.1080/01634372.2021.1920538

Bern-Klug, M., Kramer, K. W. O., Chang, G., Kane, R., Dorfman, L. T., & Saunders, J. B. (2009). Characteristics of nursing home social services directors: How common is a degree in social work? *JAMDA, 10*(1), 36–44. https://doi.org/10.1016/j.jamda.2008.06.011

Bern-Klug, M., Kramer, K. W. O., Sharr, P., & Cruz, I. (2010). Nursing home social services directors' opinions about the number of residents they can serve. *Journal of Aging & Social Policy, 22*(1), 33–52. https://doi.org/10.1080/08959420903396426

Bern-Klug, M., Smith, K. M., Roberts, A. R., Kusmaul, N., Gammonley, D., Hector, P., Simons, K., Galambos, C., Bonifas, R. P., Herman, C., Downes, D., Munn, J. C., Rudderham, G., Cordes, E. A., & Connolly, R. (2021). About a third of nursing home social services directors have earned a social work degree and license. *Journal of Gerontological Social Work*, 1–22. https://doi.org/https://doi.org/10.1080/01634372.2021.1891594

Bonifas, R. P. (2008). Nursing home work environment characteristics: Associated outcomes in psychosocial care. *Health Care Financing Review, 30*(2), 19–33.

Bonifas, R. P. (2011). Multilevel factors related to psychosocial care outcomes in Washington state skilled nursing facilities. *Journal of Gerontologicial Social Work, 54*(2), 203–223. https:// doi.org/10.1080/01634372.2010.538817

Castle, N. G. (2008). Nursing home caregiver staffing levels and quality of care: A literature review. *Journal of Applied Gerontology, 27*(4), 375–405. https://doi.org/10.1177/ 0733464808321596

Castle, N. G., & Banaszak-Holl, J. (2003). The effect of administrative resources on care in nursing homes. *Journal of Applied Gerontology, 22*(3), 405–424. https://doi.org/10.1177/ 0733464803253590

CMS. (2017). *State operations manual, appendix PP - Guidance to surveyors for long term care facilities.* Accessed August 10, 2020: https://www.cms.gov/Regulations-and-Guidance /Guidance/Manuals/downloads/som107ap_pp_guidelines_ltcf.pdf

CMS. (2020). *Design for nursing home compare five-star quality rating system: technical users' guide.* https://www.cms.gov/Medicare/Provider-Enrollment-and-Certification /CertificationandComplianc/Downloads/usersguide.pdf

Code of Federal Regulations. (2020). Title 42 (Public Health), chapter IV, subchapter G, Part 483-subpart B Section 483.70 (Administration).

Fashaw, S. A., Thomas, K. S., & McCreddy, E. (2020). Thirty-year trends in nursing home composition and quality since the passage of the omnibus reconciliation act. *JAMDA, 21*(2), 233–239. https://doi.org/org/10.1016/j.jamda.2019.07.004

Geng, F., Stevenson, D. G., & Grabowski, D. C. (2019). Daily nursing home staffing levels highly variable, often below CMS expectations. *Health Affairs, 38*(7), 1095–1100. https://doi. org/10.1377/hlthaff.2018.05322

Harrington, C., Zimmerman, D., Karon, S. L., Robinson, J., & Beutel, P. (2000). Nursing home staffing and its relationship to deficiencies. *The Journals of Gerontology. Series B,*

Psychological Sciences and Social Sciences, 55(5), S278–S287. https://doi.org/10.1093/geronb/55.5.S278

Harris-Kojetin, L. D., Sengupta, M., Lendon, J. P., Rome, V., Valverde, R., & Caffrey, C. (2019). *Long-term care providers and services users in the United States, 2015-2016*. https://stacks.cdc.gov/view/cdc/76253

Hay, K., & Chaudhury, H. (2015). Exploring the quality of life of younger residents living in long-term care facilities. *Journal of Applied Gerontology*, 34(6), 675–690. https://doi.org/10.1177/0733464813483209

Hillmer, M. P., Wodchis, W. P., Gill, S. S., Anderson, G. M., & Rochon, P. A. (2005). Nursing home profit status and quality of care: Is there any evidence of an association? *Medical Care Research and Review*, 62(2), 139–166. https://doi.org/10.1177/1077558704273769

Hox, J. (2010). *Multivariate multilevel regression models* (2nd ed.). Routledge.

Johnston, R., Jones, K., & Manley, D. (2018). Confounding and collinearity in regression analysis: A cautionary tale and an alternative procedure, illustrated by studies of British voting behaviour. *Quality & Quantity*, 52(4), 1957–1976. https://doi.org/10.1007/s11135-017-0584-6

MedPAC (Medicare Payment Advisory Commission), (2020). Medicare Payment Policy: Report to Congress. (March) http://medpac.gov/docs/default-source/reports/mar20_entire report_sec.pdf.

NASW National Association of Social Workers. (2003). *NASW standards for social work services in long-term care facilities*. https://www.socialworkers.org/LinkClick.aspx?file ticket=cwW7lzBfYxg%3D&portalid=0

Office of the Inspector General. (2003). *Psychosocial services in skilled nursing facilities*. http://oig.hhs.gov/oei/reports/oei-02-01-00610.pdf

Roberts, A. R., & Bowblis, J. R. (2017). Who hires social workers? Structural and contextual determinants of social service staffing in nursing homes. *Health & Social Work*, 42(1), 15–23. https://doi.org/10.1093/hsw/hlw058

Spanko, A. (2020). MedPAC finds total margin for nursing homes underwater for first time since 1999. *Skilled Nursing News*. (July). https://skillednursingnews.com/2020/07/medpac-finds-total-margin-for-nursing-homes-underwater-for-first-time-since-1999/

Werth, J. L., & Blevins, D. (2006). *Psychosocial issues near the end of life: A resource for professional care providers*. American Psychological Association.

Zhang, N. J., Gammonley, D., Peak, S. C., & Frahm, K. (2008-2009). Facility service environments, staffing, and psychosocial care in nursing homes. *Health Care Finance Review*, 30(2), 5–17.

Barriers to Psychosocial Care in Nursing Homes as Reported by Social Services Directors

Amy Restorick Roberts, Kevin Smith, Mercedes Bern-Klug ⓘ, and Paige Hector

ABSTRACT

This study identifies social services directors' perceptions of major barriers to psychosocial care and examines the structural factors associated with these barriers. Data were merged from the 2019 National Nursing Home Social Services Directors Survey and CMS's Nursing Home Compare. A hierarchical linear regression predicts overall barriers. Nine binary logistic regressions predict specific barriers. Common major barriers include "insufficient number of nurse aide staff" (31%), and "having to do things other people could do" (30%). Overall barriers to psychosocial care decreased as directors' years of experience increased, the number of staff members in social services increased, and less time was spent on short-stay residents. Departments with one staff member (compared to 3+) have a 300% greater likelihood of perceiving a major barrier in social services staffing, pressured discharge of short-stay residents, and residents' socioemotional needs are treated as less important than medical/nursing needs. Directors had a 59%-239% greater likelihood of perceiving a major barrier across six of the nine barriers when 50% or more of social services staffing is devoted to short-stay residents. To improve psychosocial care, federal guidelines should ensure adequate staffing levels differentiated by resident needs across short- and long-term care.

Introduction

While all nursing home staff are involved with meeting the social and emotional needs of residents, social services is uniquely responsible for providing psychosocial care (Bern-Klug & Kramer, 2013; Bonifas, 2011). Psychosocial care involves the provision of services to address the social and emotional needs of residents as they adapt to loss and change, cope with functional limitations, manage symptoms of a mental illness, and maximize self-determination and empowerment (Bonifas, 2011). Staff working in social services often have many responsibilities, including involvement with the assessment and care plan processes, advocacy of resident rights, grief support, nonpharmacological approaches to care, support for care transitions, and referrals for services (Bern-Klug & Kramer, 2013; Vourlekis et al., 2005). In an article describing quality psychosocial care, Simons et al. (2012) explain that psychosocial services should be "comprehensive in scope and address the psychological, social, emotional, and behavioral needs of residents, which can also include working closely with family members" (p. 800). These services are even more critical when residents lack an effective support system, need emotional support, experience grief and loss, or are dealing with chronic health or mental health conditions, pain, abuse of any kind, or behavioral symptoms of dementia or severe mental illness.

Psychosocial care is essential to a person's quality of life (National Association of Social Workers, 2003). In nursing homes, residents require a high level of assistance with personal care and most regulations emphasize providing an appropriate quality of care, such as administering medications, bathing, and dressing. Assessments of quality of care are typically task-oriented and intend to protect the health and safety of residents through receiving care and treatment consistent with professional standards of practice. The concept of quality of life, on the other hand, involves not only the physical aspects of care, but also the emotional and social well-being of residents along with the environmental and functional aspects of daily life within the nursing home (Kane, 2003; Shippee et al., 2015). Quality of care is a necessary, but not sufficient criteria to ensure residents' quality of life. Quality of life is assessed as a fundamental principle that applies to all care and services that each resident must receive, and facilities are required to provide the necessary care and services "to attain or maintain the highest practicable physical, mental, and psychosocial well-being" (§483.15(g)(1)).

Concerns have been raised regarding the less than optimal and inconsistent quality of psychosocial care residents receive (Kales et al., 2005; Oliver et al., 2005). National reviews highlight that despite the fact that skilled nursing facility residents had one or more psychosocial care need such as depression, anxiety, or behavioral symptoms, issues with developing appropriate care plans and following through to meet residents' social and emotional needs are prevalent (Office of the Inspector General, 2003). Furthermore, nearly half of the social services staff reported barriers to providing psychosocial care such as not having enough time, too much paperwork, insufficient social services staff, and having to do things that others could do (Office of the Inspector General, 2003). A more recent review by Levinson (2013) reported that skilled nursing facilities often fail to meet care planning and discharge planning requirements. Issues in the provision of psychosocial care are often attributed to workload and knowledge barriers (Office of the Inspector General, 2003; Parker-Oliver & Kurzejeski, 2003). There are also challenges working in an interprofessional health care teams regarding culture, self-identity, role clarification, decision-making, communication, and power dynamics (Ambrose-Miller & Ashcroft, 2016).

Advocates for improving residents' quality of life have argued that the psychosocial needs of residents should be considered equally important as the medical aspects of care, as a vital part of person-centered care practices (Zimmerman et al., 2012). The application of person-centered care within nursing homes (also known as the "Culture Change" movement led by the Pioneer Network) aims to improve quality through de-institutionalizing the traditional medical model of long-term care and honoring residents' needs and preferences by changing systems and processes to support resident direction and decision-making within a homelike atmosphere that values close relationships, staff empowerment, collaborative decision-making, and quality improvement (Koren, 2010). Integrating person-centered care involves residents and family members as well as all members of the interdisciplinary care team – including certified nursing assistants and other nursing staff, life enrichment/activities staff, food services, and more. Nurse aides, also referred to professionally as "certified nursing assistants" or "CNA's," are valuable members of the care team as they typically have the most interaction with residents on a daily basis (Harris-Kojetin et al., 2019). Due to the relationships they build with residents, CNA's are attuned to resident changes and preferences. Facilities that implement person-centered care provide better quality and have higher resident satisfaction (Grabowski et al., 2014; Poey et al., 2017).

Regulations provide guidance regarding the minimum standard of care for Medicare or Medicaid-certified nursing home facilities, although scholars agree that current regulations regarding psychosocial care should be strengthened (Bern-Klug et al., 2018; Simons et al., 2012). Weak regulations contribute to differences in facility and departmental resources and processes that affect psychosocial care delivery. For instance, the federal guidelines for the staffing levels in social services require that a facility with more than 120 beds must employ a qualified social worker on a full-time basis (§483.15(g)(2)). The staffing level requirement for a full-time "qualified social worker" is based on facility size using a cut-point of less than or more than 120 beds. Additionally, the term "qualified social worker" is very broadly defined in the guidelines as an individual with at least a bachelor's degree in social work *or a related human services* field including but not limited to sociology, special education, rehabilitation counseling, gerontology, and psychology; and at least one year of supervised social work experience in a health care setting working directly with individuals (Centers for Medicare and Medicaid Services, 2015, p. 122). The manner in which the "social worker" title is defined is inconsistent with National Association of Social Workers (NASW, 2003) guidelines that argue for "qualified social workers" to hold at least a bachelor's degree from an accredited school of social work and two years of post-graduate experience, with state licensure and credentialing by NASW. This staffing regulation focused on a facility size of less than or more than 120 beds has been criticized because it does not take into consideration resident case-mix or acuity, nor does it explain why residents in smaller facilities do not deserve to receive psychosocial care from someone with a 4-year degree (Parker-Oliver & Kurzejeski, 2003). Regardless of facility size, residents who experience similar issues such as grief and loss deserve to receive psychosocial care from a trained professional with enough time to provide person-centered care. In the literature, greater qualifications and higher staffing levels in social services are associated with better quality (Bowblis & Roberts, 2020; Roberts et al., 2020; Vongxaiburana et al., 2011).

Every facility is required to provide medically-related social services and ensure that the facility has sufficient staff who possess the basic competencies and skills to meet the behavioral health needs for residents with mental disorders, psychosocial disorders, or substance use disorders. However, most states as well as federal guidelines do not meet minimum professional social work standards for onsite psychosocial care (Bern-Klug et al., 2018). Further, different responsibilities within social services for long-term compared to short-term residents are not considered in the regulations. While both short-stay and long-stay residents require robust support, a short-stay patient typically requires intense discharge planning with varying levels of psychosocial support. For the more traditional long-term care resident, social services staff can develop a relationship to allow more discovery of person-centered needs with a comprehensive biopsychosocial-spiritual assessment and ongoing interactions to create a person-centered care plan. Directors have provided opinions about what a realistic workload should be for one full-time social services staff (20 or fewer short-stay residents or 60 or fewer long-stay residents, Bern-Klug et al., 2010). Notably, these recommendations are considerably lower than the current 120-bed federal regulation and make an argument for adjusting staffing guidelines for social services to a realistic level that is differentiated by short-stay or long-stay status, on account of the higher turnover among short-stay residents, high discharge needs, and varying degrees of biopsychosocial-spiritual needs.

Conceptual framework

In order to examine the relationship between the structure of the Department of Social Services and directors' perceptions of major barriers to psychosocial care, this study is guided by a widely-used conceptual framework for examining quality in health care settings, the Structure Process Outcome (SPO) model (Donabedian, 1966, 1988). The three categories outlined in the SPO model (Donabedian, 1966, 1988) refer to: (1) "structure" (the context and resources for care delivery such as staffing, financing, and the physical environment), (2) "process" (the way psychosocial care is delivered through interactions between residents and providers of healthcare services), and (3) "outcomes" (the effects of healthcare services that support residents' quality of life). These three components are conceptually linked in this model sequentially to propose that the structure affects process, and then process also influences quality outcomes. This model suggests that the initial focus on structure is recommended to assess and improve quality outcomes. Structure is usually more readily observable and more easily measured than the process component, and constraints or issues related to the structure of Social Services Departments may negatively impact the processes involved with psychosocial care delivery.

The first aim of the study is to identify the major barriers to psychosocial care, as reported by a national sample of social services directors. Next, drawing from the Donabedian (1966, 1988) Structure Process Outcome model, the study will examine the relationship between the structure of social services in nursing homes and major barriers to the delivery of psychosocial care. As such, the second aim of the study is to examine the association between the structure of social services (including staffing levels, the directors' educational preparedness, training, and experience, and departmental responsibilities in social services for short-term patients compared to long-term residents) and directors' perceptions of a higher number of perceived major barriers to psychosocial care. The third aim explores how the structural characteristics of social services described above are related to the likelihood of perceiving a specific major barrier.

Research design and methods

Data

This study utilized secondary data merged from the 2019 National Nursing Home Social Services Directors Survey (Bern-Klug et al., 2021) and the publicly-available Centers for Medicare and Medicaid Services (CMS) Nursing Home Compare dataset. To learn more about the study protocol, including sampling, the survey instrument, and respondent characteristics, see (Bern-Klug et al., 2021). About 30% of the directors participated in the survey (n = 924), and this study's final sample size is 808 due to the listwise deletion of missing data.

Measures

Dependent Variables: Major Barriers to Psychosocial Care
    The 2019 National Nursing Home Social Services Directors Survey (Bern-Klug et al., 2021) includes twelve items about barriers to psychosocial care previously identified through a review of the literature. Example items include "Not enough social services staff for the number of residents ... " and "social

and emotional needs are perceived as much less important than medical and nursing needs in this facility ... " From these, nine of the most commonly endorsed major barrier items to psychosocial care were included in the present study (endorsed by more than 10% of survey respondents). For each item, respondents select their level of agreement through the following four response options: not a barrier, minor barrier, moderate barrier, and major barrier (1–4). These nine items were looked at as distinct outcomes and also together as a summative score of overall barriers.

Characteristics of Social Services Departments and Directors

Guided by the SPO framework (Donabedian, 1966, 1988), variables were selected to assess the structural factors that may impact the delivery of psychosocial care. Measures for the structural aspects of social services include: staffing levels (e.g., number of workers, full-time equivalent (FTE) ratio of workers in social services to number of residents, and availability of mental health consultants), educational preparedness (e.g., training in social work, level of degree attainment, licensure/certification, the number of years of experience working in nursing home), as well as differences among positions regarding resident populations served (long-stay vs. short-stay residents). The turnover among short-stay residents is significantly higher than long-stay residents, and requires more time-intensive discharge planning work on the part of social services.

Facility Characteristics

As the organizational context may also affect the perception of major barriers to psychosocial care, the following variables were also included: facility size, location (metro, census region), ownership, resources (use of social services consultant), quality (nurse staffing levels and overall quality rating), and resident characteristics (percent of residents with severe mental illness).

Data analysis

Descriptive statistics for all study variables were examined for normality, collinearity issues, and conceptual inclusion in models. A hierarchical linear regression is used to examine whether the structural components of social services departments are related to the directors' overall perception of a higher number of major barriers to psychosocial care. Nine separate binary logistic regression models examine whether the structure of social services departments is associated with a specific barrier. The criteria to evaluate multivariate normality include skewness (+ or −2), kurtosis (+ or −6) and collinearity (e.g., VIF below 5). All analyses were conducted with SPSS 26.

Results

Descriptive statistics

In Table 1, descriptive statistics are reported for major barriers to psychosocial care and the characteristics of social services departments and facilities. On average, directors reported either a "minor" or "moderate" perceived barrier for all nine items. The most frequently reported major barriers are: insufficient number of nurse aide (CNA) staff (31%), having to do things that others could do (30%), lack of resources to provide residents opportunities to leave the nursing home on outings (25%), pressure to admit/discharge short-stay residents takes time away from attending to the social and emotional needs of long-stay residents (23%), and not enough social services staff for the number of residents (21%).

Table 1. Descriptive statistics for barriers to psychosocial care and the characteristics of social services departments and facilities (n = 924).

Major Barriers	*M* or %	*SD*	Range
Insufficient number of nurse aide staff	31%		0–1
Having to do things that others could do	30%		0–1
Lack of resources to provide residents opportunities to leave the nursing home on outings	25%		0–1
Pressure to admit/discharge short-term patients (STP)	23%		0–1
Not enough social services staff for the # of residents	21%		0–1
Staff from other departments do not consistently carry out psychosocial care plans	17%		0–1
Documentation requirements	16%		0–1
Social and emotional needs perceived as much less important than medical and nursing needs	16%		0–1
Not enough family involvement	12%		0–1
Social Services Characteristics			
Total number of workers in social services	1.67	0.88	1–4
FTE ratio in social services (# of FTE's/# residents x 100)	1.65	1.00	0–16.67
Availability of mental health consultant (No)	0.71	0.46	0–1
Education of director (1 = <4-year degree, 2 = bachelor's degree, 3 = master's degree)	2.20	0.69	1–3
Director has social work degree (Yes)	0.58	0.49	0–1
Director has social work licensure/certification (Yes)	0.47	0.50	0–1
Director's experience in NH social services (1 = <1 year, 2 = 1–3 years, 3 = 4–9 years, 4 = 10–15 years, 5 = 15+ years)	3.45	1.30	1–5
% of social services time devoted to STP (50% or more)	0.56	0.50	0–1
Facility Characteristics			
Size (120 beds or fewer)	73%		
Metro (Yes)	67%		
Census (Northeast)	16%		
Census (Midwest)	41%		
Census (South)	29%		
Census (West	14%		
Ownership (For-profit)	63%		
Use of social services consultants (Yes)	89%		
% of residents with SMI (<10% of resident population)	40%		
% of residents with SMI (10–24%)	29%		
% of residents with SMI (25–49%)	18%		
% of residents with SMI (50% or more)	13%		
Staffing (total nurse staffing)	3.84	0.84	1.69–9.12
Overall quality rating (Nursing Home Compare, 1 = 5-stars)	0.48	0.50	0–1

Notes. M = Mean, SD = Standard Deviation, STP = Short-Term Patients, MH = Mental Health, FTE = Full-Time Equivalent, NH = Nursing Home, SMI = Severe Mental Illness.

Table 2. Hierarchical linear regression for total number of barriers to psychosocial care (n = 799).

	Unstandardized		Standardized	
	B	Standard Error	β	p
Step 1	$R^2 = .059$, F = 6.239 [8, 790], $p < .001$			
Metro	−.145	.171	−.031	.395
Census Region	−.161	.085	−.068	.060
Bed Size***	.414	.121	.128	.001
For-Profit Ownership*	.426	.171	.095	.013
% Residents with SMI***	.297	.076	.143	.000
Outside SS Consultation	.343	.253	.048	.176
Quality rating (overall)	.269	.151	.062	.075
Total Nurse Staffing	−.014	.100	−.005	.889
Step 2	$R^2\Delta = .063$, FΔ = 6.956 [8, 782], $p < .001$			
Metro	−.225	.172	−.049	.191
Census Region*	−.173	.085	−.073	.042
Bed Size**	.453	.156	.141	.004
For-Profit Ownership	.317	.170	.070	.062
% Residents with SMI***	.298	.074	.143	.000
Outside SS Consultation	.270	.248	.038	.276
Quality rating (overall)	.242	.148	.056	.103
Total Nurse Staffing	.021	.104	.008	.840
Licensed/Certified	.264	.162	.061	.104
Education Level	.238	.130	.075	.067
Social Work Degree	−.042	.183	−.009	.821
Social Services FTE ratio	−.040	.097	−.018	.678
Years of Experience***	−.202	.060	−.119	.001
# of Social Services Staff*	−.235	.109	−.096	.032
Outside MH Consultation	.129	.166	.027	.438
% Time with STP***	.749	.154	.171	.000

Note. SMI = Severe Mental Illness, FTE = Full Time Equivalent, SS = Social Services, MH = Mental Health, STP = Short Term Patients.
 *$p < .05$, **$p < .01$, ***$p < .001$.

Multivariate results

The linear regression to examine the factors that contribute to directors' overall perceptions of major barriers to psychosocial care (Table 2) was fitted in two steps to separate facility-related characteristics from social services characteristics. Both steps were significant, with both steps accounting for roughly 6% of the variance, which totals 12.2% of the total variance being explained by the model. In step one, a greater number of certified beds (i.e., 60 to 120 beds or greater), for-profit ownership, and larger percentages of residents that have a severe mental illness were significantly related to a higher perception of major barriers to psychosocial care. When the social services characteristics were added in step two, the model identified that the total number of perceived major barriers to psychosocial care increased as directors' years of experience decreased, the number of staff members in social services decreased, and as directors reported a higher percentage of social services staff time devoted to short-stay residents. The overall perception of major barriers in psychosocial care also increased as census regions of nursing homes moved from the West to the East across the country, and among facilities of larger size that serve a higher percentage of residents with severe mental illness.

Next, all nine perceived major barriers to psychosocial care were examined within their own logistic regression models using the same facility and respondent characteristics (See Table 3). All models were statistically significantly different from the null hypotheses at the final step of each model (X^2 ranging between 43.70 and 98.83 with 27 dfs). Model significance was $p < .05$ for all models with five models yielding a $p < .001$ at the final model step. In addition, the major barriers of lacking social services staffing, lacking nursing aide staffing, not enough family involvement in care planning, and lacking referral resources for discharged residents were found to be significant at both the facility and social services steps of the model. Model normality was identified to fall within normative limits for all models with all Hosmer and Lemeshow Tests yielding a p value greater than 0.05. Finally, the nine models had a range of accounted for variance of 7.8% to 17.4% with "not enough family involvement" having the largest effect and "staff from other departments do not consistently carry out psychosocial care plans" having the smallest effect on variance (all reported with the Nagelkerke pseudo-R^2).

When examining the individual variable contribution across the nine logistic models, specific inferences are important to highlight. Directors reported a greater likelihood of experiencing a major barrier across six of the nine barriers when 50% or more of social services staff time is spent with short-stay residents (Odds Ratio [OR] range of 1.59 to 3.39; 59 to 239% greater likelihood). When staffed with one person (the director) there was a significantly greater likelihood of a major barrier in social services staffing needs, pressured discharge of post-acute care residents, and social and emotional needs of residents are perceived as much less important than medical and nursing needs in this facility, compared to Social Services Departments with three or more staff (all yielding an OR above 4.00; 300% greater likelihood of reporting a major barrier). However, when considering the major barrier of staff from other departments do not consistently carry out psychosocial care plans, directors with two or three staff members were significantly more likely to report this major barrier whereas directors with one staff member did not statistically differ from the reference group of three or more social services staff.

Compared to directors with 15 or more years of experience, directors with 3 years of experience or less reported increased odds (ranging between 1.93 to 5.55) of the following perceived major barriers: completing duties that could be done by others, social and emotional needs of residents are perceived as much less important than medical and nursing needs in this facility, not enough family involvement, and lack of referral resources for discharged residents (93 to 455% greater likelihood of a major barrier). Directors had a lower likelihood of reporting a major barrier when at nursing homes with

Table 3. Odds ratios from nine separate logistic regressions predicting various barriers for social services directors in U. S. nursing homes.

	Documentation Requirements	Lacking Staffing	Lacking Nurse Aides	Pressured Post-Acute Care	Lack of Care Plan Usage	Completing Others' Duties	SE Needs Less Important	Not Enough Family Involved	Lacking Resources
Metropolitan	0.90/0.82	1.17/1.11	0.78/0.72	1.02/0.85	1.35/1.27	0.86/0.78	0.87/0.81	0.68/0.81	0.91/0.83
Region: Northeast	1.08/1.01	0.78/0.70	3.21**/3.08**	1.43/1.29	1.08/0.96	1.17/1.11	1.22/1.22	1.55/1.76	1.64/1.31
Region: Midwest	1.33/1.35	0.75/0.70	2.34**/2.44**	1.36/1.30	1.43/1.26	1.32/1.31	1.28/1.06	1.74/1.57	1.17/1.02
Region: South	0.86/0.73	0.89/0.67	2.10*/1.89	1.00/0.77	1.04/0.78	0.97/0.84	1.39/1.03	1.12/1.00	1.26/0.92
Bed size: < 60	0.39*/0.32*	0.32*/0.22**	0.39**/0.49	0.72/0.68	0.70/0.75	0.68/0.72	0.79/0.66	0.32**/0.29	0.80/0.95
Bed size: 61–120	0.99/0.91	0.76/0.61*	0.47**/0.50**	0.98/0.91	0.86/0.88	0.79/0.83	0.74/0.68	0.58*/0.53	0.82/0.99
For-profit	1.03/0.89	1.26/1.16	1.56*/1.49*	0.98/0.87	1.26/1.15	1.63**/1.50*	1.21/1.07	2.39**/2.03*	1.55*/1.58*
SMI <10%	0.59/0.53*	0.56*/0.52*	0.63/0.63	0.48*/0.42**	0.77/0.76	0.82/0.79	0.58/0.57	0.22**/0.23**	0.54*/0.55*
SMI 10–24%	0.73/0.72	0.70/0.68	1.04/1.06	0.63/0.59	1.41/1.44	0.83/0.83	1.02/1.09	0.56/0.62	0.83/0.87
SMI 25–49%	0.65/0.61	0.79/0.72	1.10/1.13	0.97/0.99	1.46/1.50	1.21/1.25	0.91/0.91	0.53/0.54	0.89/0.85
SS Consultation	1.03/1.07	1.00/1.03	0.53*/0.55*	1.02/1.22	0.78/0.85	0.83/0.86	0.56/0.61	0.65/0.68	0.87/0.96
Quality rating	1.56*/1.67*	1.28/1.33	1.04/1.00	1.14/1.08	1.28/1.24	1.25/1.22	1.31/1.31	1.26/1.26	0.92/0.87
Total nurse staffing	1.11/1.13	1.09/1.17	0.77*/0.75*	1.11/1.05	0.90/0.88	1.04/1.02	1.08/1.12	1.09/1.20	0.90/0.91
Licensed/Certificate	1.23	1.26	0.86	1.1	1.53	1.08	1.76*	1.15	1.46*
Edu: <4 year degree	0.57	0.55	1	0.52	0.73	0.59	0.61	1.97	0.53
Edu: Bachelors +	0.75	0.77	0.85	0.86	0.7	0.8	0.98	1.16	0.63*
Social Work Degree	0.77	0.91	1.37	1.18	0.89	0.96	0.86	1.1	0.91
FTE ratio	0.95	0.91	0.86	1.02	0.88	0.98	0.96	0.74	0.8
Exp: <1 year	1.25	0.83	1.21	0.86	1.4	1.93*	2.07	5.55**	1.57
Exp: 1–3 years	1.26	1.23	1.39	1.13	1.58	1.39	2.88**	2.51*	1.98**
Exp: 4–9 years	0.75	0.92	1.31	1.32	1.45	1.43	1.62	1.74	1.48
Exp: 10–15 years	0.76	0.95	0.98	0.89	0.8	0.84	1.27	1.59	0.66

(Continued)

Table 3. (Continued).

Staff: 1 person	2.32	4.21**	1.03	4.51**	2.98	1.43	4.19*	1.6	0.74
Staff: 2 people	2.08	2.64*	1.04	3.10*	3.19*	1.55	3.43	1.46	0.59
Staff: 3 people	1.21	1.57	0.86	3.30*	3.50*	1.23	4.94*	1.98	0.66
MH	0.86	0.95	1.18	1.29	1.47	0.99	1	1.57	1.25
Consultation 50%+ time STP	2.00**	1.74**	1.88**	3.39**	1.49	1.66**	1.53	0.9	1.59*

Notes. Two ORs represent the 1st step OR and the second step OR (1st step/2nd step); SE = Socioemotional, SMI = Severe mental Illness, SS = Social Services, Exp = Experience, Edu = Education, MH = Mental Health, STP = Short Term Patients; Region reference = West region, Bed size reference = 121+ beds, SMI reference = 50% or greater, Edu reference = Master's degree, Experience reference = 15+ years, Staff reference = 3+ people; *p < .05, **p < .01.

fewer than 60 beds or less than 10% of residents with severe mental illness. And, directors who reported being in a nursing home with a five-star quality star rating had a greater likelihood of reporting documentation requirements as a major barrier (ORs of 1.56 & 1.67; a 56% to 67% greater likelihood).

Discussion

The first main contribution of this study is the identification of perceived major barriers to psychosocial care. The description of these barriers advances the understanding of the challenges of social services, in addition to the interaction between this department with other departments and families. Consistent with other studies that describe the demands of working in this setting (Bern-Klug & Kramer, 2013; Lee, Lee, & Armour, 2016), directors in this study reported a variety of major barriers that affect the delivery of psychosocial care. Interestingly, the most commonly reported major barrier was the insufficient number of nurse aide (CNA) staff. CNA's are vital partners in the delivery of psychosocial care, as they spend more time with residents compared to any other category of staff (Harris-Kojetin et al., 2019) and have the opportunity to get to know residents as individuals. When this knowledge is integrated into care planning and daily interactions, a true person-centered approach to care can be upheld.

The second most frequently endorsed major barrier to psychosocial care was "having to do things other people could do." Social services may spend time on tasks such as completing admissions paperwork, setting up transportation for residents to go to doctor's appointments, and finding a lost item. If the role of the social worker is not clearly delineated from a paraprofessional social services assistant (Simons et al., 2012), these and other tasks may interfere with the more clinical aspects of the director role, such as psychosocial care for residents who are dying, depressed, or experiencing a recent loss. An earlier study of directors described how social services staff "wear a lot of hats," yet have common functions (Bern-Klug & Kramer, 2013). Still, directors do report thriving in their job, a perception that is increased by higher job autonomy, being treated like an important part of the team, having enough time to identify and meet resident psychosocial needs, not having to do things that others could do, and being clear about what the role of social services is (Liu & Bern-Klug, 2013). As social services are part of interdisciplinary health care teams, directors should develop a strong sense of professional identity, clarify their role, and address power dynamics (Ambrose-Miller & Ashcroft, 2016).

A variety of major barriers to meeting psychosocial needs were reported, such as not having enough staff, documentation requirements, and pressure to admit and discharge short-stay residents which takes time away from attending to the social and emotional needs of long-stay residents. Additionally, directors identified how their ability to provide psychosocial care is reduced when staff from other departments do not consistently carry out psychosocial care plans or when families are not involved. Challenges were also reported within a facility culture where residents' social and emotional needs are perceived as much less important than medical and nursing needs in the facility, and when resources are lacking to provide residents with opportunities to leave the nursing home on outings.

While this study focused on major barriers, most directors indicated a minor or moderate barrier across all nine items, which underscores the complexity of skill required to provide holistic psychosocial care within social services, including leadership skills to promote psychosocial care across other disciplines. For culture change and person-centered care to be sustained, Zimmerman et al. (2012) argue that "every member of the interdisciplinary team must prescribe to this mindset, including administrators and supervisory staff, so that sufficient time is allowed to attend to the person, as well as the task" (p. 455). Directors should be prepared to speak up when care delivery systems are not functioning properly to advocate for the systems-level changes necessary to allow for all staff to fulfill their responsibilities and improve residents' quality of care and quality of life.

The study's second aim examines the relationship between the structure of social services and directors' overall perception of major barriers to psychosocial care. The total number of perceived major barriers to psychosocial care increases as staffing resources, such as the level of staff within the social services department and the directors' experience level decrease. Major barriers also increase with higher demands on social services staff due to the need to serve a greater number of residents, more residents with severe mental illness, and when 50% or more of overall social services staffing is spent on short-stay residents. These findings are consistent with previous studies that link higher levels of staffing and higher qualifications of social services staff with better nursing home quality (Bowblis & Roberts, 2020; Roberts et al., 2020; Vongxaiburana et al., 2011). Directors with more experience may have developed skill with setting professional boundaries, collaborating with staff in other disciplines, and leading culture change initiatives to overcome some challenges related to providing psychosocial care. In order to reduce barriers, findings support increasing the resources available to social services by ensuring adequate certified nursing assistant (CNA) staffing levels, increasing social services staffing levels, and hiring or retaining Directors of Social Services with a more nursing home experience, while considering a realistic workload to meet the psychosocial care needs of short-stay, as well as long-stay residents.

Examining the structural barriers associated with each specific challenge (aim 3) draws attention to ways in which increasing the level of social services staffing may improve aspects of psychosocial care. When the Department of Social Services is staffed by only one person (compared to three), there is a 300% greater likelihood of a perceived major barrier in staffing needs, pressured discharge of short-stay residents, and social and emotional needs of residents are treated as less important than medical and nursing needs in the facility. Although this pattern is consistent across a number of barriers, low social services staffing levels are not associated with every barrier. For instance, even departments with two or three social services staff members had a greater likelihood of reporting a major barrier of "staff from other departments do not consistently carry out psychosocial care plans," which underscores the need for the entire care team to give attention to psychosocial issues and prioritize them. Still, these findings contribute to a growing literature that illustrates how low social services staffing is related to a variety of barriers to psychosocial care and why following current federal regulations that require one full-time qualified social worker, but only for nursing homes with more than 120 beds, is problematic. In nursing homes, the issue of staffing adequacy has focused on nursing (e.g., Dellefield et al., 2015), which require minimum nursing staffing ratios. Similarly, higher minimum standards through a staffing ratio for social services would better define what constitutes a realistic caseload for social services to value the dignity of every resident, regardless of facility size.

Although federal guidelines do not require adjustments to staffing due to case-mix or resident needs, our study provides evidence of the need to differentiate social services staffing regulations based on responsibilities for short-stay versus long- stay residents. Directors reported a 59% to 239% greater likelihood of experiencing a major barrier across six of the nine barriers when the department allocates 50% or more of their staffing resources to short-stay residents. For short-stay residents, social services are often time-pressured, intensive, and include discharge planning administrative duties. The more immediate needs of short-stay residents compete with resources for long-stay residents' psychosocial care. When half or more of social services staff time is spent on short-stay residents, directors perceived major barriers related to documentation requirements, not enough social services staff for the number of residents, insufficient number of nurse aide staff (CNA's), having to do things that others could do, and a lack of resources to provide residents with opportunities to leave the nursing home on outings.

The experience level of directors also matters. Directors with three years or fewer of experience in nursing home social services (compared to directors with 15 or more years of experience) were 93% to 455% more likely to perceive major barriers in completing duties that could be done by others, socioemotional needs being less important than medical and nursing needs in the facility, not enough family involvement, and lacking referral resources for discharged residents. These findings imply that directors with more experience are better prepared to address psychosocial care needs of residents, perhaps due to stronger skills in leadership to maintain professional boundaries, collaboration with other facility directors and administration to build an organizational culture that values psychosocial care, as well as practices to encourage greater family involvement.

Some perceptions of specific major barriers are explained by facility characteristics, as well. Directors were less likely to report a major barrier to psychosocial care when the facility was small (less than 60 beds) and the facility has a low proportion of residents with severe mental illness (less than 10%). Also, the highest quality star rating facilities (5 star) have a greater likelihood of reporting the major barrier of documentation requirements.

Limitations and future research

With a focus on examining the directors' perception of major barriers to psychosocial care collectively and specifically, this study found support for a relationship between some structural aspects of social services and perceived major barriers to psychosocial care. Several limitations should be noted. First, as a cross-sectional study, the associations between the structure of social services and perceived major barriers to psychosocial care should not be interpreted as causality. Second, the dataset did not include variables to assess the "process" component of the Structure Process Outcome model (Donabedian, 1966, 1988), or other structural factors that may be related to barriers to psychosocial care, such as turnover within social services, certified nursing assistants, or administration. Relatedly, the omission of the "process" component in this study is likely responsible for why the regression models yielded a relatively low percentage of variance explained. Although other factors account for the majority of differences in directors' perceptions of major barriers in psychosocial care, the study does take a vital step forward by supporting the conceptual linkage between structure of social services and issues in psychosocial care delivery in this large, national sample of social services directors.

To build on this study, the authors recommend that research in this area includes the process component of the SPO framework (Donabedian, 1966, 1988) to understand what strategies are useful in addressing barriers to meeting the psychosocial needs of residents. Challenges in delivering psychosocial care are often related to workload and knowledge barriers (Office of the Inspector General, 2003; Parker-Oliver & Kurzejeski, 2003), thus a fuller understanding of why these issues persist could substantiate changes that may affect staffing configurations, and provide a justification for additional training and support. Research can also contribute to developing evidence-based practices for social services working with short-stay and long-stay residents. A study of how a skilled, well-trained, and adequately staffed social services department utilizes strategies to improve wellbeing, including the consideration of how much time it can take to tend to the biopsychosocial-spiritual needs of a person, would be a helpful resource. Since workers in social services must draw on a combination of skills in both direct practice and macro practice, more research to understand what personal and professional strengths align with this role may offer valuable insight in order to integrate these skills and competencies within training and social work education.

More research is needed to study how palliative care, trauma-informed care, and long-term care processes and systems used by social services staff and other disciplines may improve psychosocial care, and ultimately resident outcomes. Research could explore how interdisciplinary health care teams support a culture of person-centered care that equally values the social and emotional needs of residents as much as the medical aspects of care. In addition, social services may intervene in various ways, for example, by helping direct care workers learn about strategies to provide daily psychosocial support to residents in their care. The most frequently reported major barrier by social services directors, "insufficient number of nurse aide staff," illustrates the interdependence of adequate staffing across disciplines. Future research should holistically consider how adequate staffing across all departments in a nursing home and a care team that prioritizes psychosocial care affects resident quality of life and facility quality. Research in this area may be able to influence regulations and reimbursement models to elevate the status of psychological, social, emotional, and behavioral aspects of care.

Conclusion

This study reveals a number of challenges faced by social services, as well as the structural factors that influence the delivery of psychosocial care. Since regulations and reimbursement models strongly influence the staffing of social services in nursing homes (Roberts & Bowblis, 2017), it is critical to advocate for changing the federal regulations of the 120-bed social services staffing rule to ensure adequate staffing capacity to meet the psychosocial needs of residents. One of the largest contributions of this study demonstrates the need for higher minimum staffing standards in social services, and for these staffing levels to be differentiated based on responsibilities regarding short-stay and long- stay residents. An increased staffing level may lead to fewer perceived major barriers and ultimately better care, yet more research is need to understand the optimal social services staffing levels and configurations, as well as most promising practice approaches for interdisciplinary health care teams to overcome barriers to providing psychosocial care to improve resident and facility quality outcomes.

ORCID

Mercedes Bern-Klug (iD) http://orcid.org/0000-0001-6546-6141

References

Ambrose-Miller, W., & Ashcroft, R. (2016). Challenges faced by social workers as members of interprofessional collaborative health care teams. *Health & Social Work*, *41*(2), 101–109. https://doi.org/10.1093/hsw/hlw006

Bern-Klug, M., Byram, E., Steinberg, N. S., Garcia, H. G., & Burke, K. C. (2018). Nursing home residents' legal access to onsite professional psychosocial care: Federal and state regulations do not meet minimum professional social work standards. *The Gerontologist*, *58*(4), e260–e272. https://doi.org/10.1093/geront/gny053

Bern-Klug, M., & Kramer, K. W. O. (2013). Core functions of nursing home social service departments in the United States. *Journal of the American Medical Directors Association*, *14* (1), 75e1–75e7. https://doi.org/10.1016/j.jamda.2012.09.004

Bern-Klug, M., Kramer, K. W. O., Sharr, P., & Cruz, I. (2010). Nursing home social service directors' opinions about the number of residents they can serve. *Journal of Aging & Social Policy*, *22*(1), 33–52. https://doi.org/10.1080/08959420903396426

Bern-Klug, M., Smith, K., Roberts, A. R., Kusmaul, N., Gammonley, D., Bonifas, R., Bonifas, R., Bonifas, R., Munn, J., Munn, J., Munn, J., Cordes, E., Cordes, E., Connolly, R., & Connolly, R. (2021). About one-third of nursing home social services directors have earned a social work degree and license. *Journal of Gerontological Social Work, Available Online Ahead of Print*, 1–22. https://doi.org/10.1080/01634372.2021.1891594

Bonifas, R. P. (2011). Multilevel factors related to psychosocial care outcomes in Washington State skilled nursing facilities. *Journal of Gerontological Social Work*, *54*(2), 203–223. https://doi.org/10.1080/01634372.2010.538817

Bowblis, J. R., & Roberts, A. R. (2020). Cost-effective adjustments to nursing home staffing to improve quality. *Medical Care Research and Review*, *77*(3), 274–284. https://doi.org/10.1177/1077558718778081

Centers for Medicare and Medicaid Services. (2015). *United States Code of Federal Regulations (CRF) state operations manual (Section 42, part 483.15(g))*. Author.

Dellefield, M. E., Castle, N. G., McGilton, K. S., & Spilsbury, K. (2015). The relationship between registered nurses and nursing home quality: An integrative review (2008–2014). *Nursing Economics*, *33*(2), 95–108. http://eprints.whiterose.ac.uk/87183/

Donabedian, A. (1966). Evaluating the quality of medical care. *Milbank Quarterly*, *44*(3), 166–203. https://doi.org/10.2307/3348969

Donabedian, A. (1988). The quality of care: How can it be assessed? *Journal of the American Medical Directors Association*, *260*(12), 1743–1748. https://doi.org/10.1001/jama.1988.03410120089033

Grabowski, D. C., O'Malley, A. J., Afendulis, C. C., Caudry, D. J., Elliot, A., & Zimmerman, S. (2014). Culture change and nursing home quality of care. *The Gerontologist*, *54*(1), S35–S45. https://doi.org/10.1093/geront/gnt143

Harris-Kojetin, L., Sengupta, M., Lendon, J. P., Rome, V., Valverde, R., & Caffrey, C. (2019). Long-term care providers and service users in the United States, 2015–2016. National center for health statistics. *Vital Health Stat*, *3*(43). https://www.cdc.gov/nchs/data/series/sr_03/sr03_43-508.pdf

Kales, H. C., Chen, P., Blow, F. C., Welsh, D. E., & Mellow, A. M. (2005). Rates of clinical depression diagnosis, functional impairment, and nursing home placement in coexisting dementia and depression. *American Journal of Geriatric Psychology*, *13*(6), 441–449. https://doi.org/10.1097/00019442-200506000-00002

Kane, R. A. (2003). Definition, measurement, and correlates of quality of life in nursing homes: Toward a reasonable practice, research, and policy agenda. *The Gerontologist*, *43*(2), 28–36. https://doi.org/10.1093/geront/43.suppl_2.28

Koren, M. J. (2010). Person-centered care for nursing home residents: The culture-change movement. *Health Affairs (Project Hope)*, *29*(2), 312–317. https://doi.org/10.1377/hlthaff.2009.0966

Lee, A. A., Lee, S. N., & Armour, M. (2016). Drivers of change: Learning from the lived experiences of nursing home social workers. Social Work in Health Crae, 55(3), 1–18. DOI: 10.1080/00981389.2015.1111967

Levinson, D. (2013). *Skilled nursing facilities often fail to meet care planning and discharge planning requirements*. U.S. Department of Health and Human Services, Office of the Inspector General.

Liu, J., & Bern-Klug, M. (2013). Nursing home social services directors who report thriving at work. *Journal of Gerontological Social Work*, *56*(2), 127–145. https://doi.org/10.1080/01634372.2012.750255

National Association of Social Workers. (2003). *NASW standards for social work services in long-term care facilities*. Author.

Office of the Inspector General. (2003). Psychosocial services in skilled nursing facilities. United States Department of Health and Human Services. http://oig.hhs.gov/oei/reports/oei-02-01-00610.pdf

Oliver, D. P., Porock, D., & Zweig, S. (2005). End-of-life care in U.S. nursing homes: A review of the evidence. *Journal of the American Medical Directors Association*, *6*(3 Suppl), S21–30. https://doi.org/10.1016/j.jamda.2005.03.017

Parker-Oliver, D., & Kurzejeski, L. S. (2003). Nursing home social services. *Journal of Gerontological Social Work*, *2*(2), 37–50. https://doi.org/10.1300/J083v42n02_04

Poey, J. L., Hermer, L., Cornelison, L., Kaup, M. L., Drake, P., Stone, R. I., & Doll, G. (2017). Does person-centered care improve residents' satisfaction with nursing home quality? *Journal of the American Medical Directors Association*, *18*(11), 974–979. https://doi.org/10.1016/j.jamda.2017.06.007

Roberts, A. R., & Bowblis, J. R. (2017). Who hires social workers? Structural and contextual determinants of social services staffing in nursing homes. *Health & Social Work*, *42*(1), 15–23. https://doi.org/10.1093/hsw/hlw058

Roberts, A. R., Smith, A. C., & Bowblis, J. R. (2020). Nursing home social services and post-acute care: Does more qualified staff improve behavioral symptoms and reduce antipsychotic drug use? *Journal of the American Medical Directors Association: The Journal of Post-Acute and Long-Term Care Medicine*, *21*(3), 388–394. https://doi.org/10.1016/j.jamda.2019.07.024

Shippee, T., Henning-Smith, C., Kane, R. L., & Lewis, T. (2015). Resident- and facility-level predictors of quality of life in long-term care. *The Gerontologist*, *55*(4), 643–655. https://doi.org/10.1093/geront/gnt148

Simons, K., Bern-Klug, M., & An, S. (2012). Envisioning quality psychosocial care in nursing homes: The role of social work. *Journal of the American Medical Directors Association*, *13*(9), 800–805. https://doi.org/10.1016/j.jamda.2012.07.016

Vongxaiburana, E., Thomas, K. S., Frahm, K. A., & Hyer, K. (2011). The social worker in interdisciplinary care planning. *Clinical Gerontologist*, *34*(5), 367–378. https://doi.org/10.1080/07317115.2011.588540

Vourlekis, B., Zlotnik, J. L., & Simons, K. (2005). *Evaluating social work services in nursing homes: Toward quality psychosocial care and its measurement—A report to the profession and blueprint for action.* Institute for the Advancement of Social Work Research.

Zimmerman, S., Connolly, R., Zlotnik, J. L., Bern-Klug, M., & Cohen, L. W. (2012). Psychosocial care in nursing homes in the era of the MDS 3.0: Perspectives of the experts. *Journal of Gerontological Social Work, 55*(5), 444–461. https://doi.org/10.1080/01634372. 2012.667525

Dementia Care Involvement and Training Needs of Social Services Directors in U.S. Nursing Homes

Jung Kwak ⓘ , Kevin M. Smith, Mercedes Bern-Klug ⓘ , and Kristin Kalin

ABSTRACT

This study describes social services directors' involvement in dementia care in U.S. nursing homes, focusing on interest in and needs for dementia care training. Respondents were 924 social service directors from U.S. nursing homes. We found that 87% of social service departments engaged in cognitive assessment; 59% of social services directors were strongly interested in dementia care training, and 23% would need up to 10 hours of preparation time or would not be able to train staff on dementia-related care. Multinomial logistic regression analysis (n = 836) revealed that, in comparison to having no interest in dementia training, age, years of experience in nursing homes, outside mental health contracting, barriers to staffing, and hours needed to prepare dementia training predicted varying interest in dementia care training. These findings demonstrate social services directors' active involvement in dementia care and need for training.

Background

In 2015–2016 in the U.S., 47.8% of nursing home residents were estimated to have Alzheimer's disease or other dementias; among long-term residents, dementia prevalence was 58.9% (Harris-Kojetin et al., 2019). When persons with dementia enter nursing homes, they often have advanced needs and dementia-related behavioral symptoms, including restlessness, agitation, aggression, impaired communication, and difficulties sleeping (Brasure et al., 2016; Kales et al., 2015). The primary recommended response to these symptoms comprises a range of non-pharmacologic interventions and social care that incorporates environmental and contextual influences (Zeisel et al., 2016).

Nursing home social services directly impact residents' quality of life, especially for those living with dementia, by addressing a wide range of emotional and psychosocial needs: assistance with admission, psychosocial assessment, interpersonal challenges, decision-making support, and ensuring residents' rights. In U.S. nursing homes, social service staff are lead providers of psychosocial assessment and intervention for residents (Simons et al., 2012). Their assessment of resident needs typically includes completing psychosocial items on the Minimum Data Set (MDS), a federally mandated, standardized assessment tool for all nursing homes certified for Medicare and Medicaid payments that informs treatment planning and psychosocial care for residents (Simons et al., 2012). While all staff need to be aware of residents' psychosocial needs, social service staff are responsible for assessment and care planning and provision of psychosocial services to both residents and their family members (Roberts et al., 2020; Simons et al., 2012).

Given that many residents have cognitive impairments associated with Alzheimer's disease and other dementias, interviewing and completing comprehensive assessment as well as developing care plans for residents with cognitive limitations is a necessary component of nursing home social work practice and requires special education, training and skills (Simons et al., 2012). Moreover, the qualifications of social service staff affect resident outcomes and quality of care. Two studies of nursing homes found direct relationship between the number of qualified social service staff and psychosocial care outcomes such as reduction in behavioral symptoms and use of antipsychotic medications (Roberts et al., 2020; Zhang, Gammonley, Paek, & Frahm, 2008–2009). Social staff with more years of nursing home experience also associated with better outcomes (R. P. Bonifas, 2011b).

Yet, the educational background and preparedness of social service staff varies in part due to limited federal regulations relative to the staffing of social service professionals and broad variation in the training and credentialing of such staff at the state levels (Roberts et al., 2020; Simons et al., 2012). Furthermore, there are no federal requirements that nursing home social services staff have dementia training. A primary federal regulation in Medicare- and/or Medicaid-certified nursing homes is that those with more than 120 beds are required to employ one full-time social services staff person with a college degree related to human services. Most nursing homes employ social services staff; roughly three-fourths employ a federally "qualified social worker" (Harris-Kojetin et al., 2019).

Development of a dementia care workforce in nursing homes with more thorough training is key to quality of care and life among residents living with dementia (Weiss et al., 2020). Nevertheless, few empirical studies have examined social service staff's need for and interest in dementia-care training. In a survey of nursing home social service staff in Missouri, Parker-Oliver and Kurzejeski (2003) found that one-third lacked necessary training and support to provide high-quality services for residents. Lacey (2006) reported that social service staff had varying degrees of comfort working in end-of-life dementia care and wanted more education and training in this area. Also, R. Bonifas (2011a) found dementia care the most common area of mental health knowledge among nursing home social service staff.

In this exploratory study, using nationally representative data for social services directors in U.S. nursing homes, we explored and described the role of social services departments in dementia-related care, focusing on interest in and needs for dementia-related training among social service directors. We asked the following questions: (a) Are social service departments involved in cognitive assessment relevant to dementia care? (b) To what extent do social service directors express a need for dementia-related training? (c) What social service director and facility characteristics are associated with interest in receiving dementia care training?

Methods

Data source

Data for this study are from a 2019 survey of social services directors from a sample of U.S. nursing homes. Of the 15,578 Medicare and/or Medicaid certified nursing homes in the December 2018 Centers for Medicare and Medicaid Services (CMS) Nursing Home Compare database, a random sample of 3,650 homes were contacted to determine whether they employed social services staff. Social service directors from 3,067 nursing homes that employed social services staff were then invited to participate in the study; 924 (30%) responded. Details of this procedure are provided elsewhere (Bern-Klug et al., 2021). The study was approved by the Institutional Review Board (IRB) of the University of Iowa (IRB # 201,810,727). All potential participants received informed consent documents that explained relevant information about the study including that consent was implied by completing and returning the survey.

Measures

Dementia care involvement and training interest and needs
Of 46 tasks describing various responsibilities for nursing home social services recommended by the National Association of Social Work (NASW) and Veteran's Affairs (VA) (Simons et al., 2012), we selected one item to assess staff's involvement in cognitive assessment of residents. This item asked whether social service staff were typically involved with completing Section C (Cognitive) of the CMS Minimum data set (MDS) assessment ("yes" or "no"). The cognitive section of the MDS assessment was chosen because this assessment is directly related dementia care needs assessment and care planning. For dementia care training interest, we selected an item that asked

whether the respondent was interested in receiving training on how to instruct and support staff in psychosocial needs of persons with dementia. This item represented one of 15 topical areas for training interest in the survey. Response options were "no interest," "minor interest," "moderate interest," and "strong interest." For training needs in social service areas, respondents were asked how much time they would need to train someone else on how to compare and contrast dementia, depression, and delirium and anticipate common psychosocial needs related to cognitive loss. This item represented 1 of 27 areas for training needs assessed in the survey. Response options included "could do without prep time," "would need up to 2 hours of prep time," "would need up to 10 hours of prep time," and "not able to do at all."

Respondents' Background Characteristics

Background information Included age, gender, race (African American, Asian/Pacific Islander, Native American, White, Multi-racial, Other), educational attainment including social work degrees (bachelor's, master's, doctoral), and social work license or certification.

Barriers to care

Respondents were asked about barriers to providing social and emotional care. From 13 areas included in the survey, three items particularly relevant to social service departments' involvement in dementia care and training need were selected: "insufficient consultation or supervision," "not enough social services staff," and "not enough family involvement." Response options were "not a barrier," "minor barrier," "moderate barrier," and "major barrier."

Facilities' characteristics

In addition to survey responses, two CMS public data files provided additional data about facilities where respondents were employed (https://data.medicare. gov/data/nursing-home-compare). Facility characteristics included ownership (for profit, not-for-profit, government), location (metro vs. non-metro counties), U.S. census region (four regions), chain status (part of a chain; i.e., two or more facilities), and number of Medicare and/or Medicaid certified beds.

Data analysis

Descriptive statistics were used to assess variables for normality, collinearity, and missingness. All variables, except gender, met normality guidelines for skewness and kurtosis (e.g., normative ranges for skewness ±2 and kurtosis ±6 (Curran et al., 1996). A multinomial logistic regression model was used to determine likelihood differences between social services directors who reported no interest in dementia training and others who reported minor, moderate, or strong interest in dementia training. Collinearity was examined between study variables; no variable had a VIF above 5 (Craney & Surles, 2002). All tests for homogeneity of variance were non-significant, indicating no non-normal data within the model (Hosmer et al., 2013). Missingness was within acceptable limits; 9.5% (n = 88) of the original sample of 924 were missing for the multinomial logistic regression, leaving the total sample for regression analyses at 836. All analyses were completed with SPSS 27.

Findings

Sample Characteristics

The majority of nursing home social service directors were women (92%) and White (87%; Table 1). Almost half were licensed or certified in social work (47%), had a social work degree (46%), and had worked at least 10 years in nursing homes (47%). The majority of participants identified as female (92%) and White (88%). Most respondents were employed in nursing homes certified to accept both Medicare and Medicaid (96%) and located in metropolitan counties (67%). More respondents came from the Midwest region (41%) than from others. Data not shown in Table 1 also indicated that 54% of social services departments had only one staff person, 31% had two, and 9% had three. Nursing homes with a greater number of beds were significantly more likely to have more than one social service staff, X^2 (6, N = 911) = 210, p <.001. Only 15% of nursing homes with 60 or fewer beds employed more than one social service staff, whereas 41% of nursing homes with 60–120 beds and 76% of nursing homes with more than 120 beds employed more than one social services staff member.

Most participants (87%) responded that social service staff were involved in completing the cognitive section of the MDS assessment. The cognitive section was the third most frequently completed MDS section (after Section D, Mood, 95%, and Section Q, Participation assessment and goal setting, 91%). Twenty-three percent of respondents reported that they would need up to 10 hours of preparation time or would not be able to train other staff on residents' dementia, depression, delirium, and cognitively related psychosocial needs. Most indicated moderate (27%) or strong (59%) interest in receiving training related to the psychosocial needs of persons with dementia. Among 15 topic areas in our survey, this was the most frequently reported topic, with strong interest (data not shown). Respondents found moderate to major barriers to care to be insufficient consultation and supervision (29%), not enough social services staff (40%), and not enough family involvement (40%).

Table 1. Descriptive Characteristics of Survey Respondents ($N = 924$)

Social Service Director Characteristics (n, %)			
Gender	Male	69	7.5
	Female	845	92.1
	Diverse	3	0.3
Race	African American	56	6.2
	Asian/Pacific Islander	15	1.6
	Native American	4	0.4
	White	802	88.1
	Multi-racial	16	1.8
	Other	17	1.9
Age (years)	18–25	38	4.2
	26–34	219	24.0
	35–44	220	24.1
	45–54	213	23.3
	55–64	181	19.8
	65+	43	4.7
Years of experience in nursing home social services	<1	68	7.4
	1–3	175	19.0
	4–9	244	26.5
	10–15	147	16.0
	>15	287	31.2
Educational attainment	<BA	142	15.6
	BA/BSW	447	49.0
	MA/MSW	323	35.4
Social work degree	Yes	384	42.1
	No	528	57.9
Professional license or certification	Yes	429	47.4
	No	477	52.6
Facility Characteristics (n, %)			
Facility ownership status	For profit	572	61.9
	Government	77	8.3
	Non-profit	264	28.6
	Missing	11	1.2
Facility in metropolitan area	Metro	611	66.9
	Not metro	302	33.1
Contracts with mental health provider	Yes	810	88.8
	No	102	11.2
U.S. region	Northeast	146	16.0
	Midwest	376	41.2
	South	266	29.1
	West	125	13.7
Chain status	Not part of a chain	383	41.9
	Part of a chain of 2 + owned/leased	530	58.1
Bed size	<60	182	19.9
	60–120	483	52.9
	≥121	248	27.2
Full-time social service per resident ratio (Mean, SD)		1.7	1
Current Involvement in Dementia Care and Training Interest (n,%)			
Social services complete Cognitive section of the MDS	Yes	802	86.8
	No	122	13.2
Interest in receiving training on how you can explain and support other staff with psychosocial needs of persons with dementia	No interest	42	4.5
	Minor interest	73	7.9
	Moderate interest	253	27.4
	Strong interest	546	59.1
How much time is needed to prepare training on compare/contrast dementia, depression, and delirium and anticipate common psychosocial needs	Could do without prep time	197	21.3
	Would need up to 2 hours of prep time	486	52.6
	Would need up to 10 hours of prep time	188	20.3
	Not able to do	22	2.4
Barriers to Care (n,%)			

(Continued)

Table 1. (Continued).

Social Service Director Characteristics (*n*, %)			
Insufficient consultation/ supervision	Not a barrier	385	42.1
	Minor barrier	263	28.7
	Moderate barrier	174	19.0
	Major barrier	93	10.2
Not enough social services staff	Not a barrier	335	36.5
	Minor barrier	218	23.7
	Moderate barrier	171	18.6
	Major barrier	194	21.1
Not enough family involvement	Not a barrier	168	18.3
	Minor barrier	385	42.0
	Moderate barrier	256	27.9
	Major barrier	108	11.8

Factors associated with strong interest in dementia care

Given respondents' varying levels of interest in receiving dementia-related training, we conducted a multivariate analysis utilizing a multinomial logistic model to explore correlates of social service directors' interest in receiving training (Table 2). Level of interest in dementia training was the dependent variable with each level being in reference to respondents with no interest in dementia training. All independent variables were entered simultaneously with categorical variables as factors and the only continuous variable (i.e., full-time equivalency) as a covariate in the model. The overall model was statistically significant, $\chi^2(87) = 170.77$, $p < .001$ with pseudo-R-squared values ranging between 10.1% and 21.3% of variance accounted by the model.

In the two comparisons of minor to no interest and moderate interest to no interest, the following were significant predictors. Respondents identifying as male, being 35–54 years old (only for moderate interest) and 55 years and older, having engaged in outside mental health contracting, facing minor barriers to supervision, having minor to major barriers to staffing, and needing 2 hours or more of preparation with training for dementia needs were more likely to report an interest in dementia training than were social service directors who were female, 18–34 years old, not contacting for outside mental health, facing no barriers in supervision or staffing, and needing no time for preparation of training for dementia needs. See Table 2 for the associated odds ratios and 95% confidence intervals.

In terms of the comparison between respondents with strong interest versus no interest, significant predictors as follows. Social service directors were more likely to endorse strong interest for training in dementia-related needs when identifying as male (*OR* = 0.01), 35 years or older compared to 18–34 years old (OR = 2.33 for 34–55 years old, OR = 3.36 for 55 and up years old), having 4–9 years of experience compared to 10+ years of experience (OR = 4.70), being in a rural part of the country (OR = 2.61), engaging in outside mental health

Table 2. Multinominal Logistic Regression Predicting Likelihood of Nursing Home Social Services Directors Interest in Receiving Dementia-Related Training Compared to Having No Interest (N = 836)

	Minor Interest		Moderate Interest		Strong Interest	
	OR	95% CI	OR	95% CI	OR	95% CI
Gender (Male)	<.01***	[0.00–0.01]	<.01***	[0.00–0.01]	<.01***	[0.00–0.01]
Race (Nonwhite)	1.19	[0.18–7.78]	1.72	[0.34–8.77]	3.28	[0.68–15.86]
Age: 35–54 years	2.00	[0.61–6.55]	3.42*	[1.24–9.39]	2.33†	[0.88–6.15]
Age: 55 years and older	2.88	[0.72–11.57]	4.01*	[1.18–13.61]	3.36*	[1.03–10.89]
Experience: 1–3 years	0.53	[0.14–2.07]	1.24	[0.41–3.80]	2.41	[0.82–7.07]
Experience: 4–9 years	1.90	[0.54–6.73]	2.63	[0.84–8.23]	4.70**	[1.55–14.27]
Education <4 years of college	0.70	[0.13–3.76]	1.08	[0.25–4.69]	0.91	[0.22–3.77]
Education: Bachelor's degree	0.53	[0.18–1.54]	0.85	[0.33–2.21]	0.77	[0.31–1.95]
Social work degree	1.18	[0.42–3.36]	1.89	[0.77–4.61]	1.46	[0.62–3.46]
Licensure/certification	1.18	[0.43–3.21]	0.76	[0.32–1.81]	0.88	[0.37–2.05]
Facility ownership status	1.34	[0.50–3.61]	0.84	[0.35–2.01]	1.05	[0.45–2.47]
Rural	1.46	[0.48–4.42]	2.21	[0.84–5.82]	2.61*	[1.01–6.70]
Mental health contracting	4.29*	[1.06–17.47]	2.46*	[0.81–7.48]	2.73†	[0.93–8.00]
Census region: Northeast	0.73	[0.14–3.78]	1.11	[0.28–4.52]	0.84	[0.22–3.24]
Census region: Midwest	3.02	[0.72 12.60]	2.87†	[0.85–9.75]	1.79	[0.55–5.81]
Census region: South	1.40	[0.31–6.34]	1.66	[0.46–5.91]	1.61	[0.48–5.44]
Chain status	1.67	[0.66–4.22]	1.40	[0.62–3.16]	1.31	[0.60–2.88]
Bed size: <60	0.54	[0.16–2.54]	0.69	[0.19–2.56]	0.44	[0.12–1.53]
Bed size: 61–120	1.13	[0.37–3.46]	1.01	[0.41–2.95]	0.79	[0.30–2.06]
FTE ratio	1.01	[0.63–1.62]	1.01	[0.71–1.46]	1.14	[0.83–1.58]
Minor barriers to supervision	1.02	[0.31–3.33]	2.97*	[1.07–8.36]	2.20	[0.80–6.03]
Moderate to major barriers to supervision	0.81	[0.25–2.65]	1.05	[0.37–3.00]	1.28	[0.46–3.51]
Minor barriers to staffing	2.82†	[0.95–8.31]	2.33†	[0.91–5.98]	2.22†	[0.90–5.52]
Moderate to major barriers to staffing	11.33**	[2.66–48.27]	9.15**	[2.37–35.27]	11.56***	[3.66–43.48]
Minor barriers to family involvement	0.89	[0.29–2.78]	0.72	[0.27 1.90]	0.84	[0.33–2.17]
Moderate to major barriers to family involvement	0.96	[0.27–3.43]	0.85	[0.28–2.57]	0.95	[0.33–2.78]
Up to 2 hours of training prep needed for dementia	1.45	[0.56–3.74]	2.18†	[0.96–4.98]	2.46*	[1.11–5.44]
10+ hours or not able to do training prep for dementia needs	7.03*	[1.29–38.37]	9.70**	[1.97–47.84]	10.69**	[2.22–51.51]
Cognitive section of the MDS completed (yes)	1.09	[0.22–5.46]	0.73	[0.18–2.89]	0.54	[0.14–2.06]

Notes. UOR = Unadjusted odds ratios; CI = Confidence interval; Age reference = 18–34 years; Experience reference = 10+ years; Education reference = Master's degree; Facility ownership status reference = For profit; Census Region reference = West region; Chain status = Part of chain; Bed size reference = 121+ beds; Barriers to supervision reference = No barriers; Barriers to staffing reference = No barriers; Barriers to family involvement reference = No barriers; Time need for preparing for dementia training reference = No training prep needed. †p < .1, *p < .05; **p < .01; ***p < .001.

contracting (OR = 2.73), facing minor to major barriers to staffing compared to having no barriers (OR = 2.46 for minor barriers, OR = 11.56 for moderate to major barriers), and needing between 1 and 10+ hours, including not being able to prepare, compared to not needing any time to prepare to deliver dementia training (OR = 2.46 for up to 2 hours, OR = 10.69 for 10+ hours or unable to prep).

Discussion

Nursing home social services directly impact the quality of life of residents living with dementia, and the need for dementia care training for the nursing home workforce is a national priority (Weiss et al., 2020). In our survey, the vast majority of nursing home social services departments had completed the cognitive section of the MDS assessment, and social services directors reported greater interest in dementia care training than in any other area of training. This strong interest in dementia training was supported by almost a quarter of respondents, who reported that they would need up to 10 hours of preparation time or would not be able to train other staff on dementia, depression, delirium, and common cognitively related psychosocial needs. Competent dementia care requires knowledge of these conditions, because they can present in the same person at the same time or present separately (Simons et al., 2012). Nursing staff are keenly involved in physical care needs of residents with dementia, but social services staff must anticipate, assess, and address the psychosocial needs of persons with these multiple conditions.

In terms of respondent characteristics, respondents who were 35 years or older compared to 18–34 years old, had 4–9 years of experience compared to 10+ years of experience, and needed 1–10 hours of preparation time to deliver dementia training or were not able to prepare dementia training at all were more likely to have a strong interest in dementia training than those without these characteristics. It is understandable that social services staff less experienced with nursing home care and those who need significant amount of time to training someone on dementia care would be more interested in dementia care training. However, we are uncertain why 35 years or older participants were more interested in training than younger participants. It is possible that younger participants may be more recent graduates who received education and training on aging in general and dementia specifically, given the increasing interest in and emphasis on delivering gerontological content in both undergraduate and graduate social work and social service curricula. Future studies are warranted to examine the role of professional experience, and gerontological education and training backgrounds among different cohorts of social services directors with training interest in dementia care.

With regard to facility characteristics, the finding that a strong interest in training was associated with the facilities in a rural part of the country is consistent with the well-documented barriers to adequate staffing, funding, and training opportunities in rural health and long-term care settings. It may also be the case that in-house training opportunities may be limited in facilities that outsource mental health services and thus, explaining a strong interest in training among staff. For the association between the lack of sufficient social services staff and strong interest in training, it is plausible that nursing homes with insufficient social services staff are under-resourced for psychosocial care in general, and especially for dementia, which may lead to greater need for training and support for dementia care. Future studies may examine further and compare the availability and accessibility of and support for dementia care training for social service staff in both rural and urban areas.

In our study, we did not find any differences in the interest in dementia care training by educational attainment type and years of experience including whether the social service director had a social work degree or not. These findings suggest that while the formal dementia care education during under-graduate and or master's training is certainly important, continuing education and training for social service staff is critical to ensure high-quality dementia care delivered by social service staff. As such, more gerontological social work research is warranted to identify specific areas of knowledge and skills that social service staff with different educational and disciplinary backgrounds may have or need to develop and strengthen further in practice, and how they collaborate with other team members in delivering dementia care. Findings from such research may inform education and training efforts in development and dissemination of effective dementia care training programs for social services staff as well as development of policy to ensure adequate training and credentialing of social service staff.

Limitations of our study include its cross-sectional design, and the study was not theory-based. The survey targeted social service directors instead of all social service staff, although more than half of social services departments had only one staff person. The survey response rate was 30%, somewhat lower than the typical response rate for organizational surveys (35.7%; Baruch & Holtom, 2008). Additionally, although reasons are unknown, nursing homes in the Midwest were over-represented in our sample (41%). In the U.S., nursing homes in the Midwest represent 33% of all US nursing homes. The nature of skewness within the two predictor variables, gender and race/ethnicity, and wide confident intervals for two variables, experiencing moderate to major barriers to staffing and 10+ hours or unable to prepare to train others on dementia care suggest results should be interpreted with caution. In addition, our study finding is limited by using one-item indicators to measure dementia care involvement and training interest with limited reliability. Therefore, our results should be interpreted with caution.

To improve quality of life and effectively advocate for residents living with dementia, well-trained social services staff in essential care for persons with dementia is necessary ((Gilster et al., 2018; Roberts et al., 2020; Simons et al., 2012; Weiss et al., 2020). Our study's limitations notwithstanding, its findings from the nationally representative data for social services directors in U.S. nursing homes provide clear evidence for social services staff's involvement in dementia care and interest in and need for more dementia training. There is a strong need for more systematic efforts to develop and widely disseminate dementia care education and training for social services staff in nursing homes in the U.S.

Funding

This work was supported by the RRF Foundation for Aging (RRF# 2018-0089).

ORCID

Jung Kwak (iD) http://orcid.org/0000-0002-0635-5457
Mercedes Bern-Klug (iD) http://orcid.org/0000-0001-6546-6141

References

Baruch, Y., & Holtom, B. C. (2008). Survey response rate levels and trends in organizational research. *Human Relations, 61*(8), 1139–1160. https://doi.org/10.1177/0018726708094863

Bern-Klug, M., Smith, K.M., Roberts, A.R., Kusmaul, N., Gammonley, D., Hector, P., Simons, K., Bonifas, R., Herman, C., Downes, D., Munn, J.C., Rudderham, G., Cordes, E.A., and Connolly, R. (2021). About a third of nursing home social services directors have earned a social work degree and license. *Journal of Gerontological Social Work.* https://doi.org/10.1080/01634372.2021

Bonifas, R. (2011a). Nursing home social workers and allied professionals: Enhancing geriatric mental health knowledge. *Educational Gerontology, 37*(9), 809–832. https://doi.org/10.1080/03601271003791476

Bonifas, R. P. (2011b). Multilevel factors related to psychosocial care outcomes in Washington State skilled nursing facilities. *Journal of Gerontological Social Work, 54*(2), 203–223. PMID: 21240717. https://doi.org/10.1080/01634372.2010

Brasure, M., Jutkowitz, E., Fuchs, E., Nelson, V. A., Kane, R. A., Shippee, T., Fink, H. A., Sylvanus, T., Ouellette, J., Butler, M., & Kane, R. L. (2016). *Non-pharmacologic interventions for agitation and aggression in dementia* (Comparative Effectiveness Review No. 177). *Agency for Healthcare Research and Quality.* 177. https://www.ncbi.nlm.nih.gov/books/NBK356163/pdf/Bookshelf_NBK356163.pdf

Craney, T. A., & Surles, J. G. (2002). Model-dependent variance inflation factor cutoff values. *Quality Engineering*, *14*(3), 391–403. https://doi.org/10.1081/QEN-120001878

Curran, P. J., West, S. G., & Finch, J. F. (1996). The robustness of tests statistics to nonnormality and specification error in confirmatory factor analysis. *Psychological Methods*, *1*(1), 16–29. https://doi.org/10.1037/1082-989X.1.1.16

Gilster, S. D., Boltz, M., & Dalessandro, J. L. (2018). Long-term care workforce issues: Practice principles for quality dementia care. *The Gerontologist*, *58*(Suppl. 1), S103–S113. https://doi.org/10.1093/geront/gnx174

Harris-Kojetin, L., Sengupta, M., Lendon, J. P., Rome, V., Valverde, R., & Caffrey, C.(2019). *Long-term care providers and services users in the United States, 2015–2016* (Vital and Health Statistics Series 3, No. 43). *Centers for Disease Control and Prevention*. https://www.cdc.gov/nchs/data/series/sr_03/sr03_43-508.pdf

Hosmer, D. W., Lemeshow, S., & Sturdivant, R. X. (2013). *Applied logistic regression* (3rd ed.). Wiley.

Kales, H. C., Gitlin, L. N., & Lyketsos, C. G. (2015). Assessment and management of behavioral and psychological symptoms of dementia. *BMJ*, *350*(Article), h369. https://doi.org/10.1136/bmj.h369

Lacey, D. (2006). End-of-life decision making for nursing home residents with dementia: A survey of nursing home social services staff. *Health & Social Work*, *31*(3), 189–199. https://doi.org/10.1093/hsw/31.3.189

Parker-Oliver, D., & Kurzejeski, L. S. (2003). Nursing home social services: Policy and practice. *Journal of Gerontological Social Work*, *42*(2), 37–50. https://doi.org/10.1300/J083v42n02_04

Roberts, A. R., Smith, A. C., & Bowblis, J. R.(2020). Nursing home social services and post-acute care: Does more qualified staff improve behavioral symptoms and reduce antipsychotic drug use? *Journal of the American Medical Directors Association*, *21*(3), 388–394. https://doi.org/10.1016/j.jamda.2019.07.024

Simons, K., Connolly, R. P., Bonifas, R., Allen, P. D., Bailey, K., Downes, D., & Galambos, C. (2012). Psychosocial assessment of nursing home residents via MDS 3.0: Recommendations for social service training, staffing, and roles in interdisciplinary care. *Journal of the American Medical Directors Association*, *13*(2), 190.e9–190e15. https://doi.org/10.1016/j.jamda.2011.07.005

Weiss, J., Tumosa, N., Perweiler, E., Forciea, M. A., Miles, T., Blackwell, E., Tebb, S., Bailey, D., Trudeau, S., & Worstell, M. (2020). Critical workforce gaps in dementia education and training. *Journal of the American Geriatrics Society*, *68*(3), 625–629. https://doi.org/10.1111/jgs.16341

Zeisel, J., Reisberg, B., Whitehouse, P., Woods, R., & Verheul, A. (2016). Ecopsychosocial interventions in cognitive decline and dementia: A new terminology and a new paradigm. *American Journal of Alzheimer's Disease & Other Dementias*, *31*(6), 502–507. https://doi.org/10.1177/1533317516650806

Zhang, N. J., Gammonley, D., Paek, S. C., & Frahm, K. (2008-2009). Facility service environments, staffing, and psychosocial care in nursing homes. *Health Care Financing Review*, *30*, 5–17.

Index

accredited social work program 7, 119
activities of daily living (ADLs) 79
acute mental health symptoms 97
adjusted model 17, 18
admissions processes 46, 49, 50, 53–58
advocacy 28, 46, 47, 62, 136

Banaszak-Holl, J. 124
barriers to care 46, 158
Beaulieu, E. 48
Bern-Klug, M. 48, 63, 86
Betz, M. E. 108
biopsychosocial assessments 27, 29, 38
bivariate associations 100, 101
bivariate logistic model 16
Bonifas, R. P. 40, 47, 55, 57, 58, 131, 157

care delivery systems 148
care transitions (CT) 44–59, 75, 96, 137; social
    services involvement in 50
Carter, K. A. 63
Castle, N. G. 124
census regions 11
Centers for Medicare and Medicaid Services (CMS)
    6–8, 10, 11, 21, 22, 63, 64, 118, 119, 123, 127, 131,
    132; quality ratings 11, 14
Chaudhury, H. 122
chi-square models 87
Code of Federal Regulations 6, 7, 22, 48, 63, 116,
    118, 119
conceptual framework 139–140
continuing education 66, 71, 76, 77, 110, 164
Council on Social Work Education (CSWE) 22, 63,
    80, 118

data analysis 31, 100, 141, 158
dementia 4, 27, 40, 41, 74–76, 109, 155, 156, 158,
    159, 161, 163, 165; training 62–77, 156, 158, 161,
    163, 165
dementia care 157, 158, 161, 163–165; involvement
    and training 155–165
dependent variables 17, 18, 49, 51, 100, 126–128,
    140, 161

developing care plans 4, 30, 31, 34, 35, 39, 41, 76,
    132, 156
dichotomous variable metro/non-metro
    counties 12
disaster preparedness processes 79–91
discharge responsibilities 62–77
Donabedian, A. 140
Dupuis, S. 58

facility characteristics 7, 13–14, 29–31, 99, 101, 150,
    157, 158, 164
family involvement 41, 144, 149, 150, 159
Fashaw, S. A. 122
federal regulations 6, 7, 22, 48, 63, 76, 80, 115, 116,
    118, 119
full-time equivalent (FTE) 126

Harrington, C. 55, 124
Harris-Kojetin, L. 131
Hay, K. 122
human subjects 66

independent variables 16–18, 51, 100, 101, 107,
    127, 161
individual variables 84
individual-level structures 87
interaction analyses 18
interdisciplinary interventions 89, 96

Kurzejeski, L. S. 156

Lacey, D. 156
Levinson, D. 137
licensed social worker 4, 5, 9, 17, 18, 20, 21, 133
limitations 21, 58, 75, 89, 110, 132, 150, 164
location 81, 82, 84, 85, 99, 141, 158
logistic regression 13, 16, 31
long-term care (LTC) 46, 96, 118, 122, 123, 126,
    130, 131, 138; facilities 5, 46, 47, 97; residents
    123, 126, 128–130, 132, 133

Medicaid 7–9, 11, 13, 14, 29, 30, 48, 49, 63, 99, 116,
    122, 130; certified beds 11; funding 122

Medicare 7–9, 11, 122; funding 122;
    reimbursements 122
mental health 30, 31, 34, 39, 97–101, 110, 116, 161
moderation effects 18
multiple moderation models 16, 18
Muralidharan, A. 40

National Association of Social Workers (NASW) 5,
    6, 10, 21, 22, 47, 63, 65, 77, 80, 118, 119, 138
Nursing Home Reform Act 48, 119, 122

O'Neill, C. 55
outcome variables 49, 83, 85
ownership 9, 11, 58, 83–85, 127, 141

Parker-Oliver, D. 156
perceived competence 25, 26, 29–31, 34, 35, 37, 40;
    by resident SMI percentage 34–35
Preadmission Screening Resident Review
    (PASRR) 26
predictor variables 84, 164
psychosocial care 7, 22, 47, 98, 136, 137, 139–141,
    143, 147–151; delivery of 47, 138, 140, 141, 147,
    150, 151
psychosocial issues 4, 115, 149
psychosocial needs 27–28, 37

qualifications 53, 55, 57, 63, 97, 115, 116, 118, 133,
    139, 156
qualified social workers 5, 7, 8, 21, 22, 39, 40, 48,
    118, 119, 138
quality ratings 127

registered nurses (RNs) 11
regression model 18, 87, 150
relational factors 54–58
research design 140
resident characteristics 29, 66, 141
Roberts, A. R. 7, 39, 47, 58
rural-urban continuum codes (RUCC) 11, 12, 18,
    20, 85, 127

self-efficacy 95, 98, 100, 101, 107, 108, 110; in
    suicide risk management 100, 107
self-reported competency 101, 105
serious mental illnesses (SMI) 25–41, 109;
    percentage of residents with 30
Severe Acute Respiratory Syndrome (SARS) 109
severe mental illness 137, 141, 143, 144, 147,
    148, 150
short-stay residents 71, 139, 141–144, 147–149
Simons, K. 10, 47, 137
single-item indicators 110
skilled nursing facility (SNF) 11
skills development 108
social services (SS) 28, 31, 34, 35, 37, 40, 41, 44,
    48–50, 54, 56–58, 65, 77, 97, 100, 101, 109,

115–133, 139–141, 147–151; in planning and
    providing care 29–30; providers 26, 28, 41, 97; by
    resident SMI percentage 31–34; responsibilities
    10, 64, 68, 71; role in disaster planning 86;
    staffing 28, 63, 84, 89, 109, 128, 132, 144, 148;
    staffing ratios 8, 116, 126–132; structure of 140,
    148, 150; workforce 20, 81, 83, 97
social services departments 4, 15, 20, 29, 48, 62–64,
    86, 88, 89, 116, 141, 148, 157; characteristics 67–68
social services directors (SSDs) 3–23, 25–41, 62–64,
    76, 83, 84, 86, 87, 89, 90, 98–101, 107, 109,
    157, 161, 164; characteristics 14–16; structural
    characteristics 79–91
social services involvement 34, 35, 37, 41, 45, 50, 53,
    56, 58, 75, 76; in admissions processes 53–54; in
    care transitions 54; in disaster planning and drills 86
social services staff 5, 7, 9, 40, 62, 77, 99, 109,
    130–133, 148, 156, 157, 159, 163, 164; members
    4, 62, 63, 67, 72, 75–77, 126, 129–132
social work 4, 5, 8, 15, 20, 22, 45, 63, 77, 80, 82, 86,
    97, 118, 119, 124, 125, 138; education 8, 21, 22,
    63, 80, 90, 118, 151; in long term care 90–91;
    potential merits of 82; practice 5, 6, 8, 21, 22, 47,
    156; staffing ratios 116, 119, 123
social workers 4–6, 21, 22, 40, 41, 45–48, 57, 63,
    80, 82, 90, 97, 108, 116, 118; federal government
    rules for 6–8; professional standards for 6;
    responsibility 115; state licensure of 5
staffing 99, 108, 109, 129, 148, 149, 151, 156, 161,
    163, 164; ratios 15, 16, 22, 84, 85, 115, 123, 124,
    126, 132, 133
state laws 5, 8, 15, 21, 118
state licensure 5, 22, 138
state regulations 8–9, 74
statistical analyses 31, 50, 85, 101, 129
structural factors 54, 55, 58, 82–84, 90, 97, 101,
    150, 151
structures, nursing home 87
study limitations, SMI 40
suicide rates 95
suicide risk management 95–110
survey instrument 10, 49, 64, 66, 125, 140
Sussman, T. 58

top training priority 65, 74–76
training 40, 41, 62–65, 72, 74–76, 97, 98, 101,
    108, 125, 156, 158, 161, 163, 164; -related items
    66; interests 64, 65, 72, 157, 158, 164, 165;
    recommendations 40
transitions 4, 45, 46, 57, 96, 116

Van Orden, K. A. 109
variables 16–18, 49–51, 83, 84, 107, 125–127, 131,
    132, 158
variance inflation factor (VIF) value 128

Zimmerman, S. 148